FREE Study Skills Vide

Dear Customer,

Thank you for your purchase from Mometrix! We consider it an honor and a privilege that you have purchased our product and we want to ensure your satisfaction.

As part of our ongoing effort to meet the needs of test takers, we have developed a set of Study Skills Videos that we would like to give you for <u>FREE</u>. These videos cover our *best practices* for getting ready for your exam, from how to use our study materials to how to best prepare for the day of the test.

All that we ask is that you email us with feedback that would describe your experience so far with our product. Good, bad, or indifferent, we want to know what you think!

To get your FREE Study Skills Videos, you can use the **QR code** below, or send us an **email** at <u>studyvideos@mometrix.com</u> with *FREE VIDEOS* in the subject line and the following information in the body of the email:

- The name of the product you purchased.
- Your product rating on a scale of 1-5, with 5 being the highest rating.
- Your feedback. It can be long, short, or anything in between. We just want to know your impressions and experience so far with our product. (Good feedback might include how our study material met your needs and ways we might be able to make it even better. You could highlight features that you found helpful or features that you think we should add.)

If you have any questions or concerns, please don't hesitate to contact me directly.

Thanks again!

Sincerely,

Jay Willis
Vice President
<u>jay.willis@mometrix.com</u>
1-800-673-8175

SCAN HERE

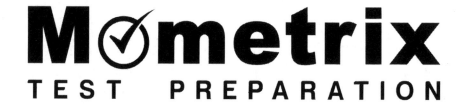

Written and edited by Mometrix Test Prep

Printed in the United States of America

This paper meets the requirements of ANSI/NISO Z39.48-1992 (Permanence of Paper).

Mometrix offers volume discount pricing to institutions. For more information or a price quote, please contact our sales department at sales@mometrix.com or 888-248-1219.

Paperback
ISBN 13: 978-1-60971-303-4
ISBN 10: 1-60971-303-6

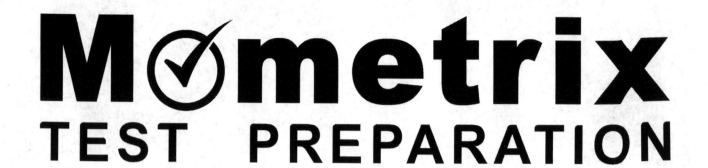

Certified Hemodialysis Technologist/Technician Exam Secrets Study Guide

CHT Test Review for the
Certified Hemodialysis
Technologist/Technician Exam

DEAR FUTURE EXAM SUCCESS STORY

First of all, **THANK YOU** for purchasing Mometrix study materials!

Second, congratulations! You are one of the few determined test-takers who are committed to doing whatever it takes to excel on your exam. **You have come to the right place.** We developed these study materials with one goal in mind: to deliver you the information you need in a format that's concise and easy to use.

In addition to optimizing your guide for the content of the test, we've outlined our recommended steps for breaking down the preparation process into small, attainable goals so you can make sure you stay on track.

We've also analyzed the entire test-taking process, identifying the most common pitfalls and showing how you can overcome them and be ready for any curveball the test throws you.

Standardized testing is one of the biggest obstacles on your road to success, which only increases the importance of doing well in the high-pressure, high-stakes environment of test day. Your results on this test could have a significant impact on your future, and this guide provides the information and practical advice to help you achieve your full potential on test day.

Your success is our success

We would love to hear from you! If you would like to share the story of your exam success or if you have any questions or comments in regard to our products, please contact us at **800-673-8175** or **support@mometrix.com**.

Thanks again for your business and we wish you continued success!

Sincerely,
The Mometrix Test Preparation Team

Need more help? Check out our flashcards at:
http://mometrixflashcards.com/BONENT

TABLE OF CONTENTS

Introduction

Thank you for purchasing this resource! You have made the choice to prepare yourself for a test that could have a huge impact on your future, and this guide is designed to help you be fully ready for test day. Obviously, it's important to have a solid understanding of the test material, but you also need to be prepared for the unique environment and stressors of the test, so that you can perform to the best of your abilities.

For this purpose, the first section that appears in this guide is the **Secret Keys**. We've devoted countless hours to meticulously researching what works and what doesn't, and we've boiled down our findings to the five most impactful steps you can take to improve your performance on the test. We start at the beginning with study planning and move through the preparation process, all the way to the testing strategies that will help you get the most out of what you know when you're finally sitting in front of the test.

We recommend that you start preparing for your test as far in advance as possible. However, if you've bought this guide as a last-minute study resource and only have a few days before your test, we recommend that you skip over the first two Secret Keys since they address a long-term study plan.

If you struggle with **test anxiety**, we strongly encourage you to check out our recommendations for how you can overcome it. Test anxiety is a formidable foe, but it can be beaten, and we want to make sure you have the tools you need to defeat it.

1

Secret Key #1 – Plan Big, Study Small

There's a lot riding on your performance. If you want to ace this test, you're going to need to keep your skills sharp and the material fresh in your mind. You need a plan that lets you review everything you need to know while still fitting in your schedule. We'll break this strategy down into three categories.

Information Organization

Start with the information you already have: the official test outline. From this, you can make a complete list of all the concepts you need to cover before the test. Organize these concepts into groups that can be studied together, and create a list of any related vocabulary you need to learn so you can brush up on any difficult terms. You'll want to keep this vocabulary list handy once you actually start studying since you may need to add to it along the way.

Time Management

Once you have your set of study concepts, decide how to spread them out over the time you have left before the test. Break your study plan into small, clear goals so you have a manageable task for each day and know exactly what you're doing. Then just focus on one small step at a time. When you manage your time this way, you don't need to spend hours at a time studying. Studying a small block of content for a short period each day helps you retain information better and avoid stressing over how much you have left to do. You can relax knowing that you have a plan to cover everything in time. In order for this strategy to be effective though, you have to start studying early and stick to your schedule. Avoid the exhaustion and futility that comes from last-minute cramming!

Study Environment

The environment you study in has a big impact on your learning. Studying in a coffee shop, while probably more enjoyable, is not likely to be as fruitful as studying in a quiet room. It's important to keep distractions to a minimum. You're only planning to study for a short block of time, so make the most of it. Don't pause to check your phone or get up to find a snack. It's also important to **avoid multitasking**. Research has consistently shown that multitasking will make your studying dramatically less effective. Your study area should also be comfortable and well-lit so you don't have the distraction of straining your eyes or sitting on an uncomfortable chair.

The time of day you study is also important. You want to be rested and alert. Don't wait until just before bedtime. Study when you'll be most likely to comprehend and remember. Even better, if you know what time of day your test will be, set that time aside for study. That way your brain will be used to working on that subject at that specific time and you'll have a better chance of recalling information.

Finally, it can be helpful to team up with others who are studying for the same test. Your actual studying should be done in as isolated an environment as possible, but the work of organizing the information and setting up the study plan can be divided up. In between study sessions, you can discuss with your teammates the concepts that you're all studying and quiz each other on the details. Just be sure that your teammates are as serious about the test as you are. If you find that your study time is being replaced with social time, you might need to find a new team.

Secret Key #2 – Make Your Studying Count

You're devoting a lot of time and effort to preparing for this test, so you want to be absolutely certain it will pay off. This means doing more than just reading the content and hoping you can remember it on test day. It's important to make every minute of study count. There are two main areas you can focus on to make your studying count:

Retention

It doesn't matter how much time you study if you can't remember the material. You need to make sure you are retaining the concepts. To check your retention of the information you're learning, try recalling it at later times with minimal prompting. Try carrying around flashcards and glance at one or two from time to time or ask a friend who's also studying for the test to quiz you.

To enhance your retention, look for ways to put the information into practice so that you can apply it rather than simply recalling it. If you're using the information in practical ways, it will be much easier to remember. Similarly, it helps to solidify a concept in your mind if you're not only reading it to yourself but also explaining it to someone else. Ask a friend to let you teach them about a concept you're a little shaky on (or speak aloud to an imaginary audience if necessary). As you try to summarize, define, give examples, and answer your friend's questions, you'll understand the concepts better and they will stay with you longer. Finally, step back for a big picture view and ask yourself how each piece of information fits with the whole subject. When you link the different concepts together and see them working together as a whole, it's easier to remember the individual components.

Finally, practice showing your work on any multi-step problems, even if you're just studying. Writing out each step you take to solve a problem will help solidify the process in your mind, and you'll be more likely to remember it during the test.

Modality

Modality simply refers to the means or method by which you study. Choosing a study modality that fits your own individual learning style is crucial. No two people learn best in exactly the same way, so it's important to know your strengths and use them to your advantage.

For example, if you learn best by visualization, focus on visualizing a concept in your mind and draw an image or a diagram. Try color-coding your notes, illustrating them, or creating symbols that will trigger your mind to recall a learned concept. If you learn best by hearing or discussing information, find a study partner who learns the same way or read aloud to yourself. Think about how to put the information in your own words. Imagine that you are giving a lecture on the topic and record yourself so you can listen to it later.

For any learning style, flashcards can be helpful. Organize the information so you can take advantage of spare moments to review. Underline key words or phrases. Use different colors for different categories. Mnemonic devices (such as creating a short list in which every item starts with the same letter) can also help with retention. Find what works best for you and use it to store the information in your mind most effectively and easily.

Secret Key #3 – Practice the Right Way

Your success on test day depends not only on how many hours you put into preparing, but also on whether you prepared the right way. It's good to check along the way to see if your studying is paying off. One of the most effective ways to do this is by taking practice tests to evaluate your progress. Practice tests are useful because they show exactly where you need to improve. Every time you take a practice test, pay special attention to these three groups of questions:

- The questions you got wrong
- The questions you had to guess on, even if you guessed right
- The questions you found difficult or slow to work through

This will show you exactly what your weak areas are, and where you need to devote more study time. Ask yourself why each of these questions gave you trouble. Was it because you didn't understand the material? Was it because you didn't remember the vocabulary? Do you need more repetitions on this type of question to build speed and confidence? Dig into those questions and figure out how you can strengthen your weak areas as you go back to review the material.

Additionally, many practice tests have a section explaining the answer choices. It can be tempting to read the explanation and think that you now have a good understanding of the concept. However, an explanation likely only covers part of the question's broader context. Even if the explanation makes sense, **go back and investigate** every concept related to the question until you're positive you have a thorough understanding.

As you go along, keep in mind that the practice test is just that: practice. Memorizing these questions and answers will not be very helpful on the actual test because it is unlikely to have any of the same exact questions. If you only know the right answers to the sample questions, you won't be prepared for the real thing. **Study the concepts** until you understand them fully, and then you'll be able to answer any question that shows up on the test.

It's important to wait on the practice tests until you're ready. If you take a test on your first day of study, you may be overwhelmed by the amount of material covered and how much you need to learn. Work up to it gradually.

On test day, you'll need to be prepared for answering questions, managing your time, and using the test-taking strategies you've learned. It's a lot to balance, like a mental marathon that will have a big impact on your future. Like training for a marathon, you'll need to start slowly and work your way up. When test day arrives, you'll be ready.

Start with the strategies you've read in the first two Secret Keys—plan your course and study in the way that works best for you. If you have time, consider using multiple study resources to get different approaches to the same concepts. It can be helpful to see difficult concepts from more than one angle. Then find a good source for practice tests. Many times, the test website will suggest potential study resources or provide sample tests.

Practice Test Strategy

When you're ready to start taking practice tests, follow this strategy:

UNTIMED AND OPEN-BOOK PRACTICE

Take the first test with no time constraints and with your notes and study guide handy. Take your time and focus on applying the strategies you've learned.

TIMED AND OPEN-BOOK PRACTICE

Take the second practice test open-book as well, but set a timer and practice pacing yourself to finish in time.

TIMED AND CLOSED-BOOK PRACTICE

Take any other practice tests as if it were test day. Set a timer and put away your study materials. Sit at a table or desk in a quiet room, imagine yourself at the testing center, and answer questions as quickly and accurately as possible.

Keep repeating timed and closed-book tests on a regular basis until you run out of practice tests or it's time for the actual test. Your mind will be ready for the schedule and stress of test day, and you'll be able to focus on recalling the material you've learned.

Secret Key #4 – Pace Yourself

Once you're fully prepared for the material on the test, your biggest challenge on test day will be managing your time. Just knowing that the clock is ticking can make you panic even if you have plenty of time left. Work on pacing yourself so you can build confidence against the time constraints of the exam. Pacing is a difficult skill to master, especially in a high-pressure environment, so **practice is vital**.

Set time expectations for your pace based on how much time is available. For example, if a section has 60 questions and the time limit is 30 minutes, you know you have to average 30 seconds or less per question in order to answer them all. Although 30 seconds is the hard limit, set 25 seconds per question as your goal, so you reserve extra time to spend on harder questions. When you budget extra time for the harder questions, you no longer have any reason to stress when those questions take longer to answer.

Don't let this time expectation distract you from working through the test at a calm, steady pace, but keep it in mind so you don't spend too much time on any one question. Recognize that taking extra time on one question you don't understand may keep you from answering two that you do understand later in the test. If your time limit for a question is up and you're still not sure of the answer, mark it and move on, and come back to it later if the time and the test format allow. If the testing format doesn't allow you to return to earlier questions, just make an educated guess; then put it out of your mind and move on.

On the easier questions, be careful not to rush. It may seem wise to hurry through them so you have more time for the challenging ones, but it's not worth missing one if you know the concept and just didn't take the time to read the question fully. Work efficiently but make sure you understand the question and have looked at all of the answer choices, since more than one may seem right at first.

Even if you're paying attention to the time, you may find yourself a little behind at some point. You should speed up to get back on track, but do so wisely. Don't panic; just take a few seconds less on each question until you're caught up. Don't guess without thinking, but do look through the answer choices and eliminate any you know are wrong. If you can get down to two choices, it is often worthwhile to guess from those. Once you've chosen an answer, move on and don't dwell on any that you skipped or had to hurry through. If a question was taking too long, chances are it was one of the harder ones, so you weren't as likely to get it right anyway.

On the other hand, if you find yourself getting ahead of schedule, it may be beneficial to slow down a little. The more quickly you work, the more likely you are to make a careless mistake that will affect your score. You've budgeted time for each question, so don't be afraid to spend that time. Practice an efficient but careful pace to get the most out of the time you have.

Secret Key #5 – Have a Plan for Guessing

When you're taking the test, you may find yourself stuck on a question. Some of the answer choices seem better than others, but you don't see the one answer choice that is obviously correct. What do you do?

The scenario described above is very common, yet most test takers have not effectively prepared for it. Developing and practicing a plan for guessing may be one of the single most effective uses of your time as you get ready for the exam.

In developing your plan for guessing, there are three questions to address:

- When should you start the guessing process?
- How should you narrow down the choices?
- Which answer should you choose?

When to Start the Guessing Process

Unless your plan for guessing is to select C every time (which, despite its merits, is not what we recommend), you need to leave yourself enough time to apply your answer elimination strategies. Since you have a limited amount of time for each question, that means that if you're going to give yourself the best shot at guessing correctly, you have to decide quickly whether or not you will guess.

Of course, the best-case scenario is that you don't have to guess at all, so first, see if you can answer the question based on your knowledge of the subject and basic reasoning skills. Focus on the key words in the question and try to jog your memory of related topics. Give yourself a chance to bring the knowledge to mind, but once you realize that you don't have (or you can't access) the knowledge you need to answer the question, it's time to start the guessing process.

It's almost always better to start the guessing process too early than too late. It only takes a few seconds to remember something and answer the question from knowledge. Carefully eliminating wrong answer choices takes longer. Plus, going through the process of eliminating answer choices can actually help jog your memory.

Summary: Start the guessing process as soon as you decide that you can't answer the question based on your knowledge.

How to Narrow Down the Choices

The next chapter in this book (**Test-Taking Strategies**) includes a wide range of strategies for how to approach questions and how to look for answer choices to eliminate. You will definitely want to read those carefully, practice them, and figure out which ones work best for you. Here though, we're going to address a mindset rather than a particular strategy.

Your chances of guessing an answer correctly depend on how many options you are choosing from.

How many choices you have	How likely you are to guess correctly
5	20%
4	25%
3	33%
2	50%
1	100%

You can see from this chart just how valuable it is to be able to eliminate incorrect answers and make an educated guess, but there are two things that many test takers do that cause them to miss out on the benefits of guessing:

- Accidentally eliminating the correct answer
- Selecting an answer based on an impression

We'll look at the first one here, and the second one in the next section.

To avoid accidentally eliminating the correct answer, we recommend a thought exercise called **the $5 challenge**. In this challenge, you only eliminate an answer choice from contention if you are willing to bet $5 on it being wrong. Why $5? Five dollars is a small but not insignificant amount of money. It's an amount you could afford to lose but wouldn't want to throw away. And while losing $5 once might not hurt too much, doing it twenty times will set you back $100. In the same way, each small decision you make—eliminating a choice here, guessing on a question there—won't by itself impact your score very much, but when you put them all together, they can make a big difference. By holding each answer choice elimination decision to a higher standard, you can reduce the risk of accidentally eliminating the correct answer.

The $5 challenge can also be applied in a positive sense: If you are willing to bet $5 that an answer choice *is* correct, go ahead and mark it as correct.

Summary: Only eliminate an answer choice if you are willing to bet $5 that it is wrong.

Which Answer to Choose

You're taking the test. You've run into a hard question and decided you'll have to guess. You've eliminated all the answer choices you're willing to bet $5 on. Now you have to pick an answer. Why do we even need to talk about this? Why can't you just pick whichever one you feel like when the time comes?

The answer to these questions is that if you don't come into the test with a plan, you'll rely on your impression to select an answer choice, and if you do that, you risk falling into a trap. The test writers know that everyone who takes their test will be guessing on some of the questions, so they intentionally write wrong answer choices to seem plausible. You still have to pick an answer though, and if the wrong answer choices are designed to look right, how can you ever be sure that you're not falling for their trap? The best solution we've found to this dilemma is to take the decision out of your hands entirely. Here is the process we recommend:

Once you've eliminated any choices that you are confident (willing to bet $5) are wrong, select the first remaining choice as your answer.

Whether you choose to select the first remaining choice, the second, or the last, the important thing is that you use some preselected standard. Using this approach guarantees that you will not be enticed into selecting an answer choice that looks right, because you are not basing your decision on how the answer choices look.

This is not meant to make you question your knowledge. Instead, it is to help you recognize the difference between your knowledge and your impressions. There's a huge difference between thinking an answer is right because of what you know, and thinking an answer is right because it looks or sounds like it should be right.

Summary: To ensure that your selection is appropriately random, make a predetermined selection from among all answer choices you have not eliminated.

Test-Taking Strategies

This section contains a list of test-taking strategies that you may find helpful as you work through the test. By taking what you know and applying logical thought, you can maximize your chances of answering any question correctly!

It is very important to realize that every question is different and every person is different: no single strategy will work on every question, and no single strategy will work for every person. That's why we've included all of them here, so you can try them out and determine which ones work best for different types of questions and which ones work best for you.

Question Strategies

READ CAREFULLY

Read the question and answer choices carefully. Don't miss the question because you misread the terms. You have plenty of time to read each question thoroughly and make sure you understand what is being asked. Yet a happy medium must be attained, so don't waste too much time. You must read carefully, but efficiently.

CONTEXTUAL CLUES

Look for contextual clues. If the question includes a word you are not familiar with, look at the immediate context for some indication of what the word might mean. Contextual clues can often give you all the information you need to decipher the meaning of an unfamiliar word. Even if you can't determine the meaning, you may be able to narrow down the possibilities enough to make a solid guess at the answer to the question.

PREFIXES

If you're having trouble with a word in the question or answer choices, try dissecting it. Take advantage of every clue that the word might include. Prefixes can be a huge help. Usually they allow you to determine a basic meaning. Pre- means before, post- means after, pro - is positive, de- is negative. From prefixes, you can get an idea of the general meaning of the word and try to put it into context.

HEDGE WORDS

Watch out for critical hedge words, such as *likely, may, can, sometimes, often, almost, mostly, usually, generally, rarely,* and *sometimes.* Question writers insert these hedge phrases to cover every possibility. Often an answer choice will be wrong simply because it leaves no room for exception. Be on guard for answer choices that have definitive words such as *exactly* and *always.*

SWITCHBACK WORDS

Stay alert for *switchbacks.* These are the words and phrases frequently used to alert you to shifts in thought. The most common switchback words are *but, although,* and *however.* Others include *nevertheless, on the other hand, even though, while, in spite of, despite, regardless of.* Switchback words are important to catch because they can change the direction of the question or an answer choice.

FACE VALUE

When in doubt, use common sense. Accept the situation in the problem at face value. Don't read too much into it. These problems will not require you to make wild assumptions. If you have to go beyond creativity and warp time or space in order to have an answer choice fit the question, then you should move on and consider the other answer choices. These are normal problems rooted in reality. The applicable relationship or explanation may not be readily apparent, but it is there for you to figure out. Use your common sense to interpret anything that isn't clear.

Answer Choice Strategies

ANSWER SELECTION

The most thorough way to pick an answer choice is to identify and eliminate wrong answers until only one is left, then confirm it is the correct answer. Sometimes an answer choice may immediately seem right, but be careful. The test writers will usually put more than one reasonable answer choice on each question, so take a second to read all of them and make sure that the other choices are not equally obvious. As long as you have time left, it is better to read every answer choice than to pick the first one that looks right without checking the others.

ANSWER CHOICE FAMILIES

An answer choice family consists of two (in rare cases, three) answer choices that are very similar in construction and cannot all be true at the same time. If you see two answer choices that are direct opposites or parallels, one of them is usually the correct answer. For instance, if one answer choice says that quantity x increases and another either says that quantity x decreases (opposite) or says that quantity y increases (parallel), then those answer choices would fall into the same family. An answer choice that doesn't match the construction of the answer choice family is more likely to be incorrect. Most questions will not have answer choice families, but when they do appear, you should be prepared to recognize them.

ELIMINATE ANSWERS

Eliminate answer choices as soon as you realize they are wrong, but make sure you consider all possibilities. If you are eliminating answer choices and realize that the last one you are left with is also wrong, don't panic. Start over and consider each choice again. There may be something you missed the first time that you will realize on the second pass.

AVOID FACT TRAPS

Don't be distracted by an answer choice that is factually true but doesn't answer the question. You are looking for the choice that answers the question. Stay focused on what the question is asking for so you don't accidentally pick an answer that is true but incorrect. Always go back to the question and make sure the answer choice you've selected actually answers the question and is not merely a true statement.

EXTREME STATEMENTS

In general, you should avoid answers that put forth extreme actions as standard practice or proclaim controversial ideas as established fact. An answer choice that states the "process should be used in certain situations, if..." is much more likely to be correct than one that states the "process should be discontinued completely." The first is a calm rational statement and doesn't even make a definitive, uncompromising stance, using a hedge word *if* to provide wiggle room, whereas the second choice is a radical idea and far more extreme.

11

BENCHMARK

As you read through the answer choices and you come across one that seems to answer the question well, mentally select that answer choice. This is not your final answer, but it's the one that will help you evaluate the other answer choices. The one that you selected is your benchmark or standard for judging each of the other answer choices. Every other answer choice must be compared to your benchmark. That choice is correct until proven otherwise by another answer choice beating it. If you find a better answer, then that one becomes your new benchmark. Once you've decided that no other choice answers the question as well as your benchmark, you have your final answer.

PREDICT THE ANSWER

Before you even start looking at the answer choices, it is often best to try to predict the answer. When you come up with the answer on your own, it is easier to avoid distractions and traps because you will know exactly what to look for. The right answer choice is unlikely to be word-for-word what you came up with, but it should be a close match. Even if you are confident that you have the right answer, you should still take the time to read each option before moving on.

General Strategies

TOUGH QUESTIONS

If you are stumped on a problem or it appears too hard or too difficult, don't waste time. Move on! Remember though, if you can quickly check for obviously incorrect answer choices, your chances of guessing correctly are greatly improved. Before you completely give up, at least try to knock out a couple of possible answers. Eliminate what you can and then guess at the remaining answer choices before moving on.

CHECK YOUR WORK

Since you will probably not know every term listed and the answer to every question, it is important that you get credit for the ones that you do know. Don't miss any questions through careless mistakes. If at all possible, try to take a second to look back over your answer selection and make sure you've selected the correct answer choice and haven't made a costly careless mistake (such as marking an answer choice that you didn't mean to mark). This quick double check should more than pay for itself in caught mistakes for the time it costs.

PACE YOURSELF

It's easy to be overwhelmed when you're looking at a page full of questions; your mind is confused and full of random thoughts, and the clock is ticking down faster than you would like. Calm down and maintain the pace that you have set for yourself. Especially as you get down to the last few minutes of the test, don't let the small numbers on the clock make you panic. As long as you are on track by monitoring your pace, you are guaranteed to have time for each question.

DON'T RUSH

It is very easy to make errors when you are in a hurry. Maintaining a fast pace in answering questions is pointless if it makes you miss questions that you would have gotten right otherwise. Test writers like to include distracting information and wrong answers that seem right. Taking a little extra time to avoid careless mistakes can make all the difference in your test score. Find a pace that allows you to be confident in the answers that you select.

KEEP MOVING

Panicking will not help you pass the test, so do your best to stay calm and keep moving. Taking deep breaths and going through the answer elimination steps you practiced can help to break through a stress barrier and keep your pace.

Final Notes

The combination of a solid foundation of content knowledge and the confidence that comes from practicing your plan for applying that knowledge is the key to maximizing your performance on test day. As your foundation of content knowledge is built up and strengthened, you'll find that the strategies included in this chapter become more and more effective in helping you quickly sift through the distractions and traps of the test to isolate the correct answer.

Now it's time to move on to the test content chapters of this book, but be sure to keep your goal in mind. As you read, think about how you will be able to apply this information on the test. If you've already seen sample questions for the test and you have an idea of the question format and style, try to come up with questions of your own that you can answer based on what you're reading. This will give you valuable practice applying your knowledge in the same ways you can expect to on test day.

Good luck and good studying!

Patient Care

Anatomy and Physiology

WATER CONTENT OF THE HUMAN BODY

The human body is largely comprised of **water**. The total body weight of an adult human is up to 60% water. The amount of water contained in the body varies with body weight. The amount of water contained in a human body is inversely related to the amount of body fat. The water contained in the body serves numerous purposes. The water contained within the cells is called intracellular fluid (ICF). It provides the medium for numerous chemical processes, such as energy production, and the metabolism of oxygen and nutrients. The water contained in the body outside the cells is called extracellular fluid (ECF). Extracellular fluid bathes the cells and protects them, and is involved in the transport of nutrients and waste. Extracellular fluid can be further divided into a number of types: interstitial fluid, intravascular fluid, and transcellular fluid.

INTRACELLULAR AND EXTRACELLULAR FLUID

Intracellular fluid accounts for approximately two-thirds of the total amount of water in the body. This is approximately 40% of the weight of the body. Intracellular fluid allows the cells to perform necessary functions.

Extracellular fluid accounts for approximately one-third of the total amount of water in the body. This is approximately 20% of the total body weight. The 3 types of extracellular fluid are found in different compartments of the body.

- The **interstitial fluid** fills the spaces between cells and surrounds the outside of the blood vessels.
- **Intravascular fluid** is found in the blood plasma.
- **Transcellular fluid** is found outside the normal compartments of the body. Transcellular fluids do not interchange easily. Examples of transcellular fluids include synovial fluid and intraocular fluid.

CREATININE

Creatinine is produced by the breakdown of creatine phosphate found in the muscle. Creatinine is produced by the body at a steady rate, and the rate of production depends on muscle mass. Creatinine is present in the blood and is filtered by the kidneys. The rate of removal by the kidneys determines blood levels of creatinine. Insufficient filtering by the kidneys leads to increased blood levels. Creatinine is not reabsorbed in the tubules to any great extent. Blood levels of creatinine are used as a measure of renal function. An increased blood level of creatinine is found only with severe damage to the nephrons. As a result, blood levels of creatinine are not useful for detecting early-stage kidney disease. The creatinine clearance test is better used to test for kidney function. Serum creatinine concentration, urine creatinine concentration, and the variables of sex, age, weight, and/or race are used to determine creatinine clearance.

SERUM CREATININE AND CREATININE CLEARANCE

Serum creatinine is measured to assess kidney function. Elderly individuals have lower levels of creatinine in the blood due to a lower muscle mass. As kidney function declines, the serum creatinine level increases. Creatinine levels normally range from 0.5-1.5 mg/dL. Diet and fluid volume do not affect serum creatinine, making serum creatinine level a useful measure of kidney function.

Creatinine clearance is defined as the volume of blood cleared of creatinine in a particular time period. Creatinine clearance is usually calculated in terms of millimeters per minute. The normal range for creatine clearance rate is 85-135 mL/min. A decrease in creatinine clearance is indicative of kidney dysfunction. The kidneys are not removing creatinine at an adequate rate.

ACID-BASE BALANCE

The acid-base balance of the body must be tightly controlled. A small change from the normal state can adversely affect many organ systems. The kidneys and lungs work together to regulate acid-base homeostasis. The levels of carbon dioxide and bicarbonate in the blood determine blood pH. The acid-base balance is obtained by regulating the levels of carbon dioxide and bicarbonate in the blood. The lungs control levels of carbon dioxide, and the kidneys regulate bicarbonate levels. By secreting and reabsorbing bicarbonate and hydrogen ions, the kidneys regulate the concentration of bicarbonate. To prevent or reverse acidosis, the kidneys secrete hydrogen ions and reabsorb bicarbonate ions. Conversely, to reverse alkalosis, the kidneys secrete bicarbonate ions and reabsorb hydrogen ions. Acidosis is easier for the body to reverse than alkalosis, because under normal conditions the human body contains bicarbonate in a concentration 20 times that of carbonic acid.

ELECTROLYTE BALANCE

Pumps located in the cell wall move **sodium** ions across the cell membrane from the interior of the cell to the exterior of the cell and transport **potassium** ions into the cell from the extracellular space. This pump is metabolically active, meaning that it requires the expenditure of energy. This mechanism allows the body to maintain different concentrations of electrolytes inside and outside the cells. Body fluids also contain nonelectrolytes, such as glucose, amino acids, nutrients, and waste products. The concentration of nonelectrolytes in body fluids is much lower than the concentration of electrolytes. Water moves across the cell membrane in both directions to balance osmolarity inside and outside the cells.

THE KIDNEYS

FUNCTION

The kidneys have numerous functions.

- The kidneys eliminate waste produced by metabolism and eliminate other toxic wastes.
- The kidneys regulate fluid volume.
- The kidneys are responsible for maintaining the balance of electrolytes.
- The kidneys regulate the pH of the blood.
- The kidneys produce renin, which affects the level of sodium, fluid volume, and blood pressure.
- The kidneys produce and secrete erythropoietin. Erythropoietin is a hormone that stimulates the bone marrow to produce red blood cells.
- The normal kidney possesses receptors for a number of different *hormones* including antidiuretic hormone (ADH), aldosterone, and parathyroid hormone. Antidiuretic hormone is produced by the pituitary gland and reduces water secretion. Aldosterone is produced and secreted by the adrenal cortex. It causes the body to retain sodium. Parathyroid hormone increases the secretion of phosphorus and bicarbonate.

ANATOMY

A kidney is bean-shaped and concave on its medial aspect. The hilum is found in the concave portion of each kidney. The **hilum** is the entry site for a number of structures including the renal artery, renal vein, nerves, and ureter. The kidney is covered by a capsule of fibrous tissue and connective tissue. The **renal cortex** of the kidney is directly under this capsule. Inside the cortex is the **renal medulla**. The renal medulla is divided to form 10-20 **renal pyramids**. A renal pyramid and the renal cortex that overlies it form a **renal lobe**. The **papilla** is the tip of the renal pyramid. Each papilla drains into a **minor calyx**. A collection of minor calyces work together and drain into a **major calyx**. The major calyces drain into the **renal pelvis**. From the renal pelvis, urine exits through the **ureter** to the urinary bladder.

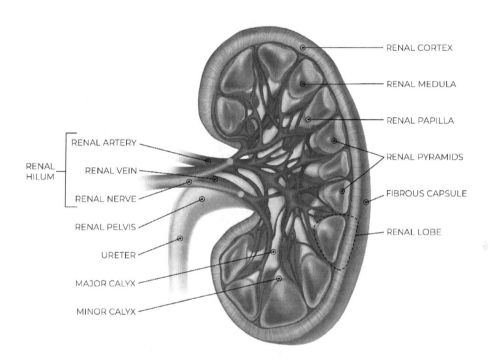

POSITION

A single kidney weighs approximately 150 g. The approximate dimensions of the kidney are as follows: length, 10 cm; width, 5.5 cm; and thickness, 3 cm. The kidneys are located in the **posterior portion of the abdominal cavity.** There is a kidney located on either side of the spinal column. The right and left kidneys are positioned slightly differently in the abdominal cavity. The right kidney is slightly lower than the left and is located just under the liver. The left kidney is situated more medially than the right. It sits under the diaphragm beside the spleen. The two adrenal glands are located above the kidneys. The kidneys sit even with the 12th and 13th thoracic vertebrae. These retroperitoneal organs are partially protected by the 11th and 12th ribs. They are covered and protected by 2 layers of fat. These layers of fat are called perirenal and pararenal fat.

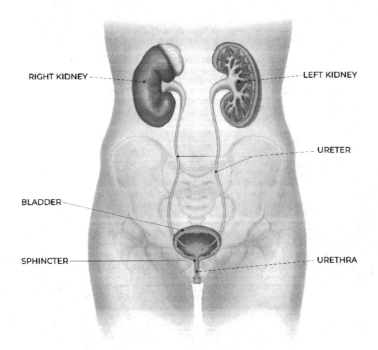

THE NEPHRON

The nephron is the unit of the kidney that is responsible for filtering and purifying the blood. It is a tube that is closed at one end and open at the other. One to two million nephrons are found in the cortex of each kidney. A nephron is made up of a vascular component and a tubular component. The vascular component of the kidney is comprised of the afferent arteriole, glomerulus, efferent arteriole, and peritubular capillaries. The tubular component of a nephron consists of Bowman's capsule, proximal tubule, loop of Henle, and the distal tubule. The nephron helps maintain homeostasis. For example, the nephron regulates the levels of water, salts, glucose, and urea in the body. The nephron is the structure that is responsible for the resorption of water and salts.

BLOOD SUPPLY

The kidneys have an **extensive network of blood vessels**. Twenty percent to twenty-five percent of the total cardiac output is directed to the kidneys. This amounts to more than 1000 mL of blood per minute. Each kidney has a separate blood supply. The renal arteries are short blood vessels that branch off from the abdominal aorta. The blood enters each kidney through a renal artery. The renal artery branches and creates the afferent arterioles. The afferent arterioles branch to form the glomerular capillaries that are found in each of the glomeruli. The glomerular capillaries then connect to create the efferent arterioles. The blood then flows from the efferent arterioles into the peritubular capillaries and the vasa recta. Blood exits each kidney through a renal vein.

THE RENAL CORPUSCLE

The renal corpuscle may also be referred to as the Malpighian corpuscle and the Malpighian body, although these terms are no longer commonly used. The renal corpuscle is the initial filtering mechanism in the kidney. It consists of Bowman's capsule and the glomerulus (below). Bowman's capsule is located at the closed end of the tube forming the nephron. The pushed-in end of the tube forms a double-walled chamber called Bowman's capsule. Bowman's capsule is a cup-shaped structure made of epithelia. The space between the layers of Bowman's capsule is continuous with the proximal tubule. The glomerulus is a network of capillaries contained within Bowman's capsule. The capillaries are supplied blood by an afferent arteriole.

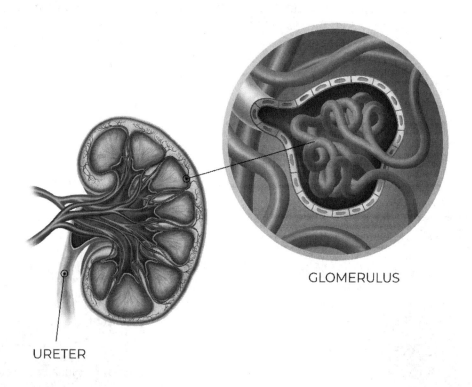

GLOMERULUS

URETER

URINE PRODUCTION

Blood enters the kidney at the hilus through the renal artery. The renal artery branches inside the cortex of the kidney and surrounds the nephrons. Blood enters the glomerulus through an afferent arteriole. The blood is filtered as it passes through the capillary walls. Water, together with dissolved solutes (albumin), flow through into Bowman's capsule. The fluid is called glomerular filtrate, and it is almost protein-free. The rate of production of the glomerular filtrate is called the **glomerular filtration rate (GFR).** GFR is a measure of the volume of filtrate produced by the kidneys every minute. A minimum level of blood circulation to the glomerulus is necessary for normal glomerular filtration. The rate of filtration decreases with increasing molecular weight and size. Because the basement membrane of the glomerulus carries a net negative charge, any substance with a negative charge will be repelled and will not be filtered.

UREA

Urea is a waste product found in urine and produced by the metabolism of protein. The amount of urea in the urine can be used to measure the breakdown of protein in the body. This is called the urine urea nitrogen test. All urine excreted is collected over a period of 24 hours. Normal values of urea in the urine range from 6-17 g over a 24-hour collection period, or 60-90 mg/dL of urine. The test can be used to assess protein balance, protein intake, and kidney function. Abnormally low levels of urea may indicate an insufficient level of protein in the diet, increased resorption, or kidney dysfunction. A high level of urea may indicate too much protein in the diet, or an increased rate of protein metabolism.

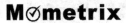

MOVEMENT OF FILTRATE THROUGH THE TUBULES

The renal tubules serve to reabsorb and secrete substances. Resorption involves the movement of filtrate back into the bloodstream via the peritubular capillaries and the vasa recta. From Bowman's capsule, filtrate travels through the proximal convoluted tubule where the glucose, sodium, amino acids, and water in the filtrate are reabsorbed. The filtrate then continues through the loop of Henle. After passing through the loop of Henle, the filtrate moves through the distal convoluted tubules. The sodium level is adjusted in the collecting tubules. The urine becomes more concentrated as it progresses through the renal tubule system. Most resorption takes place in the proximal convoluted tubule, but the distal convoluted tubule does play a role. The tubules also secrete such substances as potassium, hydrogen, ammonia, and creatinine. The blood is now filtered and leaves the kidney via the renal vein.

HORMONES THAT IMPACT THE KIDNEYS

RENIN-ANGIOTENSIN SYSTEM

Long-term blood pressure is controlled by the renin-angiotensin system (RAS), also called the renin-angiotensin-aldosterone system (RAAS). The RAS is activated by a drop in blood volume or blood pressure. Sodium ions are reabsorbed in the distal convoluted tubules. Aldosterone, a hormone, increases the rate at which this occurs. Renin, an enzyme, is released by the distal convoluted tubules of the kidneys when blood pressure becomes too low. This enzyme then converts angiotensinogen, a blood protein, to angiotensin I. Angiotensin I is then transformed by the angiotensin-converting enzyme (ACE) into angiotensin II in the capillaries of the lungs. At this point, angiotensin II stimulates secretion of aldosterone by the adrenal cortex. Aldosterone acts on the renal tubules, causing an increase in the resorption of sodium ions. This results in an increase in water volume. This volume of blood is ultimately increased, raising blood pressure.

ALDOSTERONE AND ANTIDIURETIC HORMONE (ADH)

Aldosterone is a steroid hormone produced and secreted by the zona glomerulosa in the cortex of the adrenal gland. This hormone's actions on the distal convoluted tubules and collecting ducts of the kidney regulate sodium and potassium levels in the body. Aldosterone controls the conservation of sodium through resorption and causes the secretion of potassium. The regulation of these electrolytes by aldosterone helps maintain normal blood pressure. Abnormally high levels of aldosterone can lead to hypertension, muscle cramps, and muscle weakness.

Antidiuretic hormone (ADH), also called arginine vasopressin, is secreted by the posterior pituitary gland. ADH helps regulate the concentrations of water and solutes. An antidiuretic reduces the volume of water in the urine, thereby conserving water. Antidiuretics reduce the amount of urine excreted. Large amounts of ADH cause the production of concentrated urine and cause nausea, vomiting, muscle cramps, seizures, and confusion.

ATRIAL NATRIURETIC HORMONE

Atrial natriuretic hormone (ANH) is also called atrial natriuretic peptide (ANP), and atrial natriuretic factor (ANF). It acts on the kidney as a vasodilator and reduces the resorption of sodium in the renal tubules. It helps maintain homeostasis by lowering water and sodium levels in the body. It is also involved in the homeostatic regulation of adiposity. Atrial natriuretic hormone is stored in the atria of the heart in muscle cells called atrial myocytes. These cells are stretch receptors. Atrial natriuretic hormone is released by these cells in response to hypervolemia, exercise, and calorie restriction. Atrial natriuretic hormone reduces blood pressure by reducing water, sodium, and adipose levels in the body. ANH acts to counter the actions of the renin-angiotensin system, which increases blood pressure and blood volume.

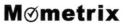

Evaluating Fluid Management

REPLACEMENT THERAPY

HEMODIALYSIS

Hemodialysis is a process by which the blood is cleared of toxins, extra fluid, extra salts, and metabolic waste products. The blood flow is directed through a semipermeable membrane that filters out these substances. A few ounces of blood at a time are directed through the semipermeable membrane. The toxins, salts, fluids, and waste products are transported away in the dialysis fluid. The cleaned blood is then returned to the body. Healthy kidneys perform this function, and hemodialysis is used when the kidneys are unable to adequately filter the blood. Hemodialysis helps regulate blood pressure and maintain electrolyte balance in the body. The dialysis treatment is prescribed individually for each patient.

CONTINUOUS RENAL REPLACEMENT THERAPY (CRRT)

Continuous renal replacement therapy (CRRT) is used to treat acute kidney injury. The technique is used particularly in the treatment of patients with multiple organ failure. Patients with acute kidney injury and multiple organ failure are usually hemodynamically unstable and exhibit cardiac insufficiency. These patients may not tolerate hemodialysis well, whereas CRRT is a slower filtration process which has less impact on hemodynamic stability.

Some procedures involving continuous renal replacement therapy require arterial access. In these procedures it is possible that the artery will be damaged, and there is risk of hemorrhage. Hemorrhage can occur if the blood circuit leaks or if one or more of the access connections are faulty. If the patient is hypotensive, the blood flow rate may not be adequate for effective filtration to occur. Clotting problems often occur with this type of therapy. If the technique being used uses venous flow, a blood pump is necessary, as air may be taken into the blood circuit.

SLOW CONTINUOUS ULTRAFILTRATION (SCUF)

Slow continuous ultrafiltration (SCUF) is a technique for removing fluid gradually that does not significantly change the levels of solutes in the body. Hemodialysis may be necessary on an intermittent basis to treat azotemia and maintain normal electrolyte levels. In a 24-hour period, SCUF can usually remove 2-6 liters of fluid.

Protein breakdown is a common occurrence in patients with acute kidney injury. For this reason, these patients may need infusions of large amounts of parenteral nutrition fluid. A normal hemodialysis treatment may not remove enough fluid to compensate for this. SCUF can be used to remove the excess fluid on a continuous basis.

EQUIPMENT NEEDED AND POSSIBLE PROBLEMS

SCUF requires a highly permeable hemofilter. The hemofilter works much like a dialyzer. A blood pump is not needed with SCUF, but it may be used. The patient's cardiac output and mean arterial pressure can provide enough pressure to move blood across the filter at an adequate rate. The ultrafiltrate is pushed through the membrane by the hydrostatic pressure of the blood. The ultrafiltrate then flows into a drainage bag. The drainage bag is disposed of after treatment. A tube runs between the hemofilter and the fluid collection device. This setup creates negative pressure that drives the rate of ultrafiltration.

The main problem with SCUF is an insufficient ultrafiltration flow rate. This may be caused by kinked tubing, clot formation in the hemofilter, reduced blood flow through the circuit, or a decrease in arterial pressure.

CONTINUOUS ARTERIOVENOUS HEMOFILTRATION (CAVH)

Continuous arteriovenous hemofiltration (CAVH) is used to remove fluid and serum solutes via the extracorporeal circuit over a prolonged time period. CAVH is performed using hemofilters designed for the purpose. The hemofilters come in a variety of sizes. CAVH is appropriate for use when the patient is hemodynamically unstable and requires large amounts of fluid removed. The removal of large amounts of fluid also allows for the removal of solutes by convection. In adults, the volume of fluid removed by CAVH is generally in the range of 8-15 L a day. A blood pump is not necessary when CAVH is used. The patient's blood pressure must be adequate to force the blood through the circuit. The mean arterial pressure must exceed 60 mmHg. The ultrafiltrate is collected in a drainage bag attached to the filter.

CONTINUOUS ARTERIOVENOUS HEMODIALYSIS (CAVHD)

CAVHD combines ultrafiltration and dialysis and is a modified version of CAVH. It removes fluid and solutes by both dialysis and ultrafiltration. The dialysis portion uses diffusion, and the ultrafiltration portion uses convection. CAVHD is used when CAVH does not remove waste products adequately. CAVHD may be a more appropriate treatment choice than CAVH if the patient is anuric, hyperkalemic, or acidotic. CAVH and CAVHD differ in one important way. In CAVHD the dialysis fluid is made to circulate around the hemofilter membrane. This results in the more efficient removal of urea and creatinine from the blood. The dialysis fluid used in CAVHD may be peritoneal dialysis fluid or a custom dialysis fluid. Custom dialysis fluid may be used to prevent hyperglycemia and lactic acidosis. It may also be used if the patient has liver failure.

CONTINUOUS VENOVENOUS HEMOFILTRATION (CVVH)

CVVH is a modified version of CAVH. It is a continuous therapy that utilizes a blood pump to regulate the flow of blood through the hemofilter. As this is a therapy involving the veins, the access is provided through the subclavian, internal carotid, or femoral veins. Solutes in the blood are removed by convection. Fluid is removed by use of ultrafiltration. Replacement fluid is administered before or after filtration to maintain the volume in the vascular system. The composition of the replacement fluid varies depending on the patient's needs. This treatment is appropriate for use with patients who cannot tolerate the rapid removal of fluids and rapid changes in solute concentrations.

INDICATIONS

CVVH is appropriate for use in hemodynamically unstable patients that require the removal of large volumes of fluid. CVVH is the treatment of choice for patients with acute kidney injury and cardiovascular instability. The technique is also appropriate for burn patients and patients with cardiogenic shock, increased intracranial pressure, shock, and multi-organ failure. CVVH uses blood pump equipment. This is advantageous when the patient's blood pressure is not sufficient to drive the extracorporeal circuit. The blood pump allows higher rates of blood flow, and this allows a higher rate of ultrafiltration and urea clearance. Because of the increased blood flow due to the pump, there is less risk of clotting in the hemofilter. CVVH can remove solutes of larger molecular weight because the hemofilter is more porous.

CONTINUOUS VENOVENOUS HEMODIALYSIS (CVVHD)

Continuous venovenous hemodialysis (CVVHD) is a continuous renal replacement treatment that uses a blood pump to regulate the flow of blood. It uses a venovenous access system. In the CVVHD system, the dialysis fluid runs against the flow of blood through the extracorporeal circuit. This requirement differs from CVVH and CVVHD. CVVHD is used for the same populations of patients as CAVHD. This treatment is appropriate for patients who are clinically unstable and cannot physically tolerate a more aggressive form of hemodialysis. The treatment is used for patients who need more therapy than intermittent hemodialysis can provide. It is used in critically ill patients with acute kidney injury who experience multiple organ failure.

SUSTAINED LOW-EFFICIENCY DIALYSIS (SLED)

SLED, also called **extended daily dialysis**, is used in the treatment of acute kidney injury. The treatment involves the administration of dialysis over an extended period of time. The dialysis treatment may last 8-12 hours. The blood flow rate in SLED is equal to, or less than, 200 mL/min. The dialysate flow rate is 100-300 mL/min. SLED provides hemodynamic stability. SLED can be administered as an alternative to intermittent hemodialysis therapy. The desired level of ultrafiltration can be obtained because of the hemodynamic stability conferred by SLED. The treatment is appropriate for patients who are critically ill. SLED is becoming an increasingly popular mode of treatment for acute kidney injury.

SHORT DAILY DIALYSIS AND INTERMITTENT NOCTURNAL IN-CENTER DIALYSIS

Short daily dialysis involves a regimen of 2-hour sessions conducted 6 or 7 times a week. Short daily dialysis is a rapid and intense form of treatment. Patients on short daily dialysis report better health and take fewer medications than patients receiving dialysis in a facility. Patients on short daily dialysis have fewer dietary restrictions and fewer fluid restrictions.

In intermittent nocturnal in-center dialysis, the patient dialyzes at a dialysis facility 3 nights a week. Each treatment lasts 8 hours. The blood and flow rates are lower in this type of dialysis than in traditional dialysis. The treatment is gentler than traditional dialysis, and the risk of hypotension and other complications is reduced. The patient is able to carry on with his or her normal daytime activities. This method produces superior clearance.

DAILY NOCTURNAL HEMODIALYSIS

Nocturnal hemodialysis is a type of home hemodialysis. The patient dialyzes at night while he or she is sleeping. The dialysis regimen is 7-10 hours a night for 6 or 7 nights each week. Because longer periods of dialysis are possible with nocturnal hemodialysis, blood flows can be reduced to approximately 200 mL/min and dialysate flows can be decreased to 300 mL/min. The patient on nocturnal hemodialysis may be monitored by dialysis staff through an internet connection. If problems occur, an alarm sounds, alerting the dialysis staff. Proper action can then be taken. This type of daily dialysis is associated with better health and the need for fewer medications. Nocturnal hemodialysis on a daily basis is a very efficient way to remove particles of larger molecular weight. Because of the frequency of the dialysis treatments, nightly nocturnal hemodialysis resembles normal kidney function.

REMOVAL OF SUBSTANCES DURING DIALYSIS

The **temperature** of the dialysis solution (dialysate) influences solute removal. The higher the dialysate temperature, the more solutes are removed from the blood. **Blood flow rate** also affects removal of solutes. Greater rates of blood flow result in greater rates of solute removal. The **molecular weight of the solutes** in the blood is related to their clearance rate. Smaller solutes are more easily removed from the blood. The **concentration gradient** during dialysis affects removal of solutes. Greater concentration gradients lead to greater levels of diffusion. The **membrane permeability** used in dialysis also influences the removal of solutes. A more permeable membrane allows more solutes to be filtered from the blood.

TYPES OF SUBSTANCES REMOVED

Generally, if a substance can be excreted by the kidneys, it will be removed by dialysis. If a substance is broken down in the liver, it will not necessarily be removed by hemodialysis. Many common substances are removed easily by dialysis. These include propylene glycol (antifreeze), ethylene, acetylsalicylic acid (aspirin), and lithium carbonate. Emergency hemodialysis therapy is also required to treat patients who have ingested certain toxic mushrooms. Prompt treatment for the ingestion of toxins with hemodialysis can prevent damage such as blindness, renal failure, and liver necrosis. An overdose of some therapeutic drugs may be administered by accident. These medications include antibiotics, theophylline, and mannitol. Emergency treatment with dialysis is required. In case of poisoning, a dialyzer with the largest possible surface area is needed. This will rid the body of the toxic substance as rapidly as possible. Dialyzers that will clear molecules of 500-20,000 Da are appropriate.

DIALYSIS IN SPECIAL POPULATIONS

CHILDREN

Children on hemodialysis may experience pain or discomfort when the needle is inserted into the fistula. Pain on insertion of the needle can be managed with the use of topical anesthetics or subcutaneous lidocaine (1% solution) injected at the insertion site. Not all children experience pain relief from topical anesthetics and many children object to the lidocaine injection. For these children, it may be best to simply insert the dialysis needle without the use of an anesthetic. **Pain management techniques,** such as imagery and deep breathing, may be used to good effect. It may be necessary to immobilize the child to insert the dialysis needle. In this case, as few personnel as possible should be involved. The personnel immobilizing the child should prevent the child's joints from moving. If the child weighs less than 10 kg, swaddling is the best option for immobilization. Restraints should only be used when absolutely necessary.

ELDERLY PATIENTS

Elderly patients may benefit from the socializing possible at a dialysis facility. Patients can be monitored by trained personnel and this may permit the early diagnosis and treatment of complications. Shorter treatment sessions are possible with hemodialysis than with peritoneal dialysis. Elderly patients on hemodialysis are more likely to experience hemodynamic instability than younger dialysis patients. Cardiac arrhythmias and hypotensive episodes are more likely in elderly patients. Hemodynamic instability can usually be reduced in severity, and even prevented, if appropriate methods are employed. Some patients may experience significant stress during the trips to and from the dialysis facility. If their complications are no more severe than those of younger patients, elderly patients may do just as well on hemodialysis.

COMORBIDITIES IN ELDERLY PATIENTS

Older patients with end-stage renal disease are likely to have **comorbidities**. The presence of comorbid conditions can make the management of end-stage renal disease more difficult. Examples of comorbidities found among older patients with end-stage renal disease include cardiovascular conditions, osteoporosis, nutritional deficiencies, impaired pulmonary function, cognitive dysfunction, impaired mental ability, and impaired mobility.

Trial dialysis is dialysis prescribed for a defined period of time to determine if the patient can benefit from the treatment. If the outcome of dialysis is in question, trial dialysis may be recommended. The duration of the trial period and the goals of the treatment are decided prior to the initiation of treatment. If the goals are not reached, the treatment is discontinued at the end of the trial period.

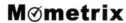

HEMODIALYSIS CONCEPTS
CONCENTRATION GRADIENT

The solution used in dialysis contains electrolytes, and it is similar in make up to plasma water. Water molecules, electrolytes, and other types of small particles can pass through the dialysis membrane in both directions. If the concentration of a particular molecule is higher on one side of the membrane, this particle will pass through to the side with lower concentration through the process of diffusion. The concentration of certain particles in the dialysate is lower than the concentration of these same particles in the blood. The difference is defined as the **concentration gradient**. The concentration gradient makes dialysis possible. The solutes move from the area of high concentration in the blood to an area of lower concentration in the dialysate. There will only be a net flow of solutes from the blood to the dialysate if the concentrations of these solutes are higher in the blood.

MASS TRANSFER RATE

The transport of undesired and/or excess solute across a semipermeable membrane from an area of high concentration to an area of low concentration is called mass transfer. The rate at which this movement occurs is called the mass transfer rate. Mass transfer rate is also referred to as solute flux. There are a number of factors that affect mass transfer rate. The mass transfer rate varies during the dialysis treatment as it is affected by these factors. If the temperature is kept constant, mass transfer rate is influenced by the solute concentration gradient and the dialyzer's physical characteristics. The characteristics of the dialyzer include the effective membrane surface area, the permeability of the membrane, the flow rates of the blood and fluid, and flow geometry.

FLOW GEOMETRY

Flow geometry is an important concept in the administration of dialysis treatment that refers to the direction in which the blood and dialysate flow. The blood and dialysate (dialysis fluid) may flow in the same direction, or may flow in opposition directions. Countercurrent flow refers to a situation in which the blood flows in one direction, and the dialysate flows in the opposite direction. This flow geometry creates the most efficient concentration gradient. Concurrent flow refers to a situation in which the blood and dialysate flow in the same direction. This situation is less than optimum, as the concentration gradient it creates is much smaller.

DIFFUSIVE TRANSPORT

Diffusive transport, also called conductive transport, is a term describing the movement of solute particles through the dialysis membrane from the side with the higher concentration of solutes to the side with the lower concentration of solutes.

The rate of diffusive transport is affected by a number of factors. The speed of diffusive transport is affected by the concentration gradient of the solutes involved. The surface area of the dialysis membrane affects speed of transport across the membrane. The rate of diffusive transport increases with increasing surface area. The mass transfer coefficient for each solute depends on the characteristics of the dialysis membrane. For thinner membranes and for more porous membranes, the mass transfer coefficient is greater as the solutes pass through more easily. The mass transfer coefficient also depends on the rates at which the blood and dialysate flow.

SIEVE COEFFICIENT AND CONVECTIVE TRANSPORT

The size of the solute particles relative to the size of the pores of the dialysis membrane affects the ease with which the particles pass through the pores. If the pore to particle ratio is high enough so that particles can pass through the pores without restriction, the **sieve coefficient** is stated to be 1. If all the particles are too large to pass through the pores, then the sieve coefficient is stated to be 0.

25

Convective transport occurs because of negative pressure on the dialysate side of the membrane (dialysate compartment) and positive pressure on the blood side of the membrane (blood compartment). This creates a net hydrostatic pressure gradient between the two compartments. Because of this hydrostatic pressure gradient, water and solutes flow from the blood compartment to the dialysate compartment. Convective transport is the transfer of solutes brought about by this process.

IMPORTANCE OF CONVECTIVE TRANSPORT

Particles may have a low sieve coefficient and low diffusive transport. In this case, the convective component becomes a major part of the total transfer of these particles. High-flux hemodialysis, hemodiafiltration, and hemofiltration are convective treatments. These methods are considered to be superior to standard diffuse hemodialysis. Convective treatments use high-flux semisynthetic and synthetic dialysis membranes. These membranes are highly permeable and permit water and electrolytes to be removed by convection.

FLOW RATE AND CLEARANCE

Clearance is a measurement of kidney function. It refers to the volume of blood that is completely cleared of a specific substance in a set period of time. Clearance is stated in terms of mL/min. Clearance deals with a theoretical volume and not a real volume of blood. The clearance of small molecules varies with the flow rate of the dialysis fluid. Urea is a solute that is affected by dialysate flow rate. Dialysate flow rate is usually 500 mL/min. Some types of dialyzers may use slower flow rates. A slower dialysate flow rate results in lower clearance of urea. High-efficiency dialyzers use faster flow rates to achieve a higher clearance of urea. The flow rate used with a high-efficiency dialyzer may exceed 500 mL/min. A higher dialysate flow rate can be used to compensate for a slower blood flow rate. Blood flow rate may be adjusted for clinical reasons, and dialysis fluid flow rate can be adjusted accordingly.

ULTRAFILTRATION

Ultrafiltration is a type of filtration that works by hydrostatic pressure. Plasma fluid is pushed out of the blood compartment, through the semipermeable membrane, and into the dialysate compartment by the hydrostatic pressure gradient. The difference in hydrostatic pressure between the 2 compartments affects the speed at which the fluid is removed. Water and solute particles of low molecular weight pass through the membrane while solute particles of high molecular weight are retained in the blood compartment. The force of pressure needed to push fluid through a membrane is called the transmembrane potential. It is the membrane's pressure gradient. Modern dialyzers generally use a combination of positive pressure in the blood compartment and negative pressure in the fluid compartment.

SEQUENTIAL ULTRAFILTRATION

Sequential ultrafiltration involves the use of ultrafiltration on its own, before the actual dialysis treatment is started. During the ultrafiltration phase of sequential ultrafiltration, the patient's blood goes through the dialyzer as normal, but the dialysate does not circulate through the dialyzer at this time. The fluid resulting from this process is collected and measured. A greater volume of fluid can be removed by this process than by conventional ultrafiltration. Sequential ultrafiltration does not cause hypotension. The process is useful in treating patients with consistently large gains in fluid.

ISOLATED ULTRAFILTRATION

Isolated ultrafiltration involves the removal of excess fluid without significantly changing the concentrations of solutes in the blood. Urea and creatinine are removed from the blood in very small amounts. This is a passive removal. The volume of extracellular fluid, the volume of fluid in the vascular system, and the stability of the patient's cardiovascular system determine the amount of fluid that can be removed.

Isolated ultrafiltration is appropriate when fluid must be removed, but the removal of solutes is not of immediate concern. Isolated ultrafiltration is a technique that can be used before hemodialysis, after hemodialysis, or individually without hemodialysis. Complications are due to the fact that, in isolated ultrafiltration, fluid is removed rapidly, and this can cause low blood pressure and cramping of the muscles.

ULTRAFILTRATION PROFILING

Ultrafiltration profiling allows the dialyzer to be set to remove different amounts of fluid at predetermined times during a single treatment. There are a number of profiles that can be used. Each profile removes a predetermined total volume of fluid, but each profile removes this fluid on a different schedule. In one profile, the dialyzer may be set to remove the largest volume of fluid during the first half of the treatment. This is the time when more fluid is present. During the second half of the treatment, the dialyzer is set to remove a smaller volume of fluid. At this time, there is less fluid left to refill the vascular space. Other ultrafiltration profiles can be used and the profile is selected according to the patient's needs.

IMPACT OF HYDROSTATIC PRESSURE

The blood and fluid flow rate during dialysis depends on the particular dialyzer in question and the transmembrane pressure of the semipermeable membrane. The transmembrane pressure is the pressure gradient of the dialysis membrane. When a new dialyzer is being used, the ultrafiltration coefficient must be determined. The ultrafiltration coefficient is different for every dialyzer. To determine the ultrafiltration coefficient, the average ultrafiltration rate per mmHg transmembrane pressure is determined. The ultrafiltration coefficient is expressed as k_{uf}. This stands for the mL/hr of fluid cleared for each mmHg. Higher k_{uf} values reflect the ability to clear greater volumes of fluid with less pressure to the semipermeable membrane of the dialyzer.

CONTROL OF ULTRAFILTRATION

Ultrafiltration is controlled by equipment designed for this purpose. There are 2 types of systems used to control ultrafiltration. These are the volumetric (balancing) system, and the servo-feedback (flow sensor) system.

- The **volumetric system** uses pumps to balance inflow to the fluid compartment and outflow from the fluid compartment. This creates a closed loop. A separate pump designed to remove fluid from this closed loop is part of the system. The operator of the dialyzer can set this pump to remove fluid at the desired rate.
- The **servo-feedback system** makes use of flow meters to monitor dialysis inflow (Q_{di}) and dialysis outflow (Q_{do}). This information is fed into a microprocessor that subtracts Q_{di} from Q_{do} to keep track of the rate of filtration (Q_{uf}). The dialyzer operator sets the ultrafiltration rate. The microprocessor adjusts the TMP accordingly to achieve the desired result.

OPERATION OF VOLUMETRIC ULTRAFILTRATION DEVICES

The volumetric ultrafiltration device is the most advanced system for ultrafiltration control. The outflow and inflow of the dialysis fluid is balanced by the actions of diaphragm chambers or double-gear systems. This volumetric ultrafiltration device ensures that the volume of fluid entering the dialyzer is equal to the volume of fluid leaving the dialyzer. A separate line branches off from the dialysate outflow line. This separate line enters an ultrafiltration pump which is controlled by a central computer processor. The ultrafiltration pump and the central computer processor control the rate of ultrafiltration. The central computer processor monitors the programmed ultrafiltration and the total ultrafiltration and makes adjustments as needed. The branch line to the ultrafiltration pump rejoins the dialysate outflow pathway before the fluid is sent to the drain.

OPERATION OF FLOWMETRIC ULTRAFILTRATION CONTROL SYSTEM

The flowmetric system is a type of ultrafiltration controller. It regulates the volume of fluid leaving the dialyzer, the volume entering the dialyzer, and the volume of ultrafiltrate. The flowmetric ultrafiltrate control system is comprised of either 1 or 2 flow meters located in the dialysate pathways entering and leaving the dialyzer. These flow meters monitor the volume of fluid in the inflow pathway and in the outflow pathway. An electronic control module regulates the speed of the pump in the outflow dialysis pathway. This ensures that the volume of dialysis fluid passing through the outflow meter is equal to the volume of dialysis fluid passing through the inflow meter plus the desired amount of ultrafiltrate.

SODIUM MODELING

Ultrafiltration can cause various physical problems. Sodium modeling, also called sodium variation, can be used to prevent dialysis-associated hypotension and cramping. Hypotension can occur as a result of dialysis treatment. It occurs because plasma fluid is taken out of the intravascular space during ultrafiltration. With rapid dialysis, the fluid from the extravascular space cannot refill the intravascular space quickly enough to prevent hypotension. Hypotension occurs with a deficit in plasma volume. In addition, the extremities may cramp because of the lack of sufficient perfusion when the vascular volume is depleted. The sodium variation system (SVS) was designed to speed up the vascular refill during ultrafiltration. Ultrafiltration involves a computer model of the movement of sodium and water between the dialysate and blood compartments during dialysis.

TECHNIQUES

In sodium modeling, the amount of sodium contained in the dialysate is manipulated during the dialysis treatment. More often, the sodium concentration in the dialysate is decreased (referred to as a decreasing profile) during treatment (though alternating and increasing profiles are also used). This can be accomplished in 2 ways. An infusion pump can be used to introduce a special sodium chloride (NaCl) concentrate to the dialysate. The proportions of substances in the usual dialysis fluid can be varied as the dialysis procedure proceeds. The sodium concentration is raised or lowered with minor changes in the levels of other electrolytes.

HIGH-FLUX DIALYSIS

High-flux dialysis requires a special dialyzer. The high-flux dialyzer has a highly permeable membrane composed of a synthetic material. Both small and larger molecular-weight solutes can cross the membrane by convection. The membrane used in high-flux dialysis can clear solutes ranging from a molecular weight of 5000 to 12,000 Da. The surface area of a membrane used in high-flux dialysis is 0.6-2.0 m². The water permeability of high-flux membranes is higher than that of a high-efficiency membrane or conventional membranes. High-flux membranes have a k_{uf} of 20-80 mL/hr per mmHg. Ultrafiltration control is necessary. The blood flow rate in a high-flux system is 300-500 mL/min. The flow of dialysis fluid is 500-800 mL/min. It is necessary to use bicarbonate dialysate. The use of high-quality water is particularly important with a high-flux system due to membrane permeability.

FUNCTIONING OF THE HIGH-FLUX DIALYZER

A high rate of dialysate flow, a high rate of blood flow, and an exact control of ultrafiltration volume is necessary for the proper functioning of the high-flux dialyzer. Synthetic membranes with a very high permeability are used with high-flux dialyzers. Solute transport is achieved in large part by convective transfer. This type of dialyzer has an ultrafiltration coefficient of at least 20-70 mL/hr per mmHg. The dialysate pressure profile produced by the ultrafiltration controller causes a reverse filtration. The reverse filtration involves the reversal of flow from the dialysis fluid to the blood in the distal section of the dialyzer. This reverse flow results in contamination when pyrogenic material and endotoxin fragments enter the blood. This contamination occurs because the membranes used in high-flux dialysis allow the passage of larger particles.

HIGH-EFFICIENCY DIALYSIS

High-efficiency dialysis is a procedure that allows the removal of larger solutes than is possible with conventional dialysis. Solutes of low to middle molecular weights can be removed. It can remove molecules of up to 5000 Da. A special dialyzer is used with a large surface area. In high-efficiency dialysis, the k_{uf} is 5-15 mL/hr per mmHg. This system requires an ultrafiltration control system to prevent excessive fluid loss in the patient. High-efficiency dialysis places the patient at higher risk of cardiovascular instability. The rapid removal of fluid can result in hypotension. A bicarbonate delivery system is necessary to maintain the stability of the cardiovascular system while still permitting fluid removal. The rate of blood flow using high-efficiency dialysis ranges from 300-500 mL/hr. The flow of dialysis fluid ranges from 500-1000 mL/hr.

EQUIPMENT NEEDED

High-efficiency dialysis requires particular equipment. There are four **equipment requirements** for high-efficiency dialysis:

- A cellulose membrane that is **highly permeable** is necessary. This membrane must have a surface area of at least 1.5 m^2. Examples of acceptable cellulose membranes include ultrathin Cuprophane, Hemophan, and cellulose acetate ester.
- There must be a **consistent blood flow** of at least 350 mL/min. The flow of the dialysis fluid must be at least 750 mL/min.
- The dialysis unit must have a delivery system that can use bicarbonate dialysate.
- The dialysis unit must have an **ultrafiltration control system**. This system offers enhanced small molecule, intermediate-size molecule, and large molecule transfer rates.

Collecting and Evaluating Patient Data

PREPARING THE PATIENT FOR THEIR FIRST DIALYSIS TREATMENT

Before the first dialysis, the physician evaluates the patient and writes the dialysis prescription. A nurse should determine the type of dialyzer to be used based on the patient's prescription. A consent form for dialysis treatment is obtained, and this record is placed in the patient's medical record. The patient's physical condition is assessed. This includes taking vital signs and weighing the patient. The nurse should ask the patient questions about his or her general health, renal functioning, and bowel functioning. The patient's fluid status is assessed. At the first dialysis treatment, the details of the treatment are determined. For the first dialysis treatment, the physician usually prescribes a 2-hour dialysis treatment with a slow blood flow.

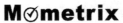

PRE-DIALYSIS QUESTIONS REGARDING PREVIOUS TREATMENT

When the hemodialysis technician is carrying out the **pre-dialysis assessment** of weight, vital signs, and general evaluation, the hemodialysis technician should question the patient to determine if any problems or events occurred since the previous treatment:

- Have you had any hospitalizations or visits to an urgent care facility or emergency department?
- How has your appetite been? Any nausea or vomiting?
- Have you had any diarrhea or other bowel problems?
- Have you had a change in medications or dosages?
- Have you taken any medications today before coming for treatment?
- Have you experienced any unusual bleeding or bruising?
- Do you have pain anywhere?
- Have you experienced any episodes of light-headedness, dizziness, or fainting?
- Are you passing any urine? How much? How frequently?
- Do you have any questions about your treatment or condition?
- Have you experienced any changes in mood or mental status?
- What is your fluid intake since the last treatment?
- How much sodium/salt do you usually have in your diet?
- Have you had any falls since your last treatment?

PRE-ASSESSMENT PROCEDURE

At the pre-assessment, the patient's health is assessed. The patient's fluid status is assessed. To this end, the respiratory rate and effort are determined, the patient is checked for jugular vein distension, and the lungs and heart are auscultated. The patient is examined for signs of edema. The patient is weighed, and his or her blood pressure is taken while sitting and standing. The total physical response (TPR) is evaluated. The patient's skin color, turgor, and integrity are assessed. The patient's temperature is taken. The patency of the vascular access is determined and the access is checked for bleeding and infection. The results of the patient's physical examination are interpreted and all precautions and necessary intervention is taken.

VITAL SIGNS

Vital signs are taken at the start of dialysis to serve as a baseline for later assessment of the patient's health. Vital signs include temperature, pulse, and respiration. An elevated temperature in a dialysis patient is indicative of an infection or illness that could complicate the patient's condition. For example, an elevated temperature may mean that that patient has a vascular access infection, or it could be a reaction to pyrogen contamination. A high dialysis fluid temperature can raise the patient's temperature. Anemia or fluid overload can cause the pulse to increase. Arrhythmia can indicate a cardiac condition. Ultrafiltration can cause a decrease in blood volume, which leads to an increase in pulse rate. The increase in pulse rate may be followed by a rapid decrease in blood pressure. An undesirable level of fluid gain may be indicated by an increase in the rate of breathing.

BLOOD PRESSURE

Blood pressure is often a result of the volume of fluid contained in the body. If a dialysis patient is hypertensive, it may indicate too much fluid in the body. Hypotension may be indicative of too little fluid in the body or dehydration. The patient's blood pressure must be measured while he or she is standing and while he or she is sitting. This is to determine if there are orthostatic changes that require intervention. In a patient with end-stage renal disease, it is the trend in blood pressure, rather than the individual readings, that is important. If the systolic blood pressure value of an end-stage renal disease patient is higher than 170 mmHg, or less than 90 mmHg, there is reason for concern. If the diastolic value is greater than 100 mmHg, this is also a reason for concern.

SITES WHERE BLOOD PRESSURE MAY BE TAKEN

The following considerations must be made when selecting the site to take a blood pressure reading:

- **Contraindications**: Never obtain blood pressure in a limb containing an access, as damage results. If both arms contain access, use thigh measurements. If there is femoral access in addition to upper arm access, use the ankle.
- **Equipment**: Incorrect cuff size makes readings inaccurate. The cuff bladder width must exceed patient's arm diameter by 20% or more. Use a thigh cuff or a bariatric cuff on the upper arm for obese patients. Use a pediatric cuff for children or adults with thin arms.
- **Arm Method**: 1. Fit the cuff to the upper arm with the bottom edge 1" above elbow joint. 2. Hold the stethoscope over the brachial artery at the elbow bend. 3. Elevate the arm after positioning the cuff, but before inflating it, to decrease venous congestion. 4. Inflate the cuff to 180 mmHg, then slowly release the air at 2-3 mmHg/sec for an accurate reading. 5. Record first Korotkoff sound heard as systolic pressure. 6. Record last Korotkoff sound heard during cuff deflation as diastolic pressure.
- **Thigh Variation**: 1. Fit the thigh cuff on the mid-thigh. 2. Hold stethoscope over popliteal artery at knee bend. Repeat steps 4 through 6 from above.
- **Ankle Variation**: 1. Fit arm cuff on ankle. 2. Hold stethoscope over dorsalis pedis artery or posterior tibial artery. Repeat steps 4 through 6 from above.
- **Charting**: Always document site used on treatment flow sheet, including the side (left or right). Not note, leg pressures are 20-40 mmHg higher than arm readings.

HEART SOUNDS

Heart sounds should be auscultated prior to and following each dialysis session. The lub-dub sound signals one cardiac cycle or heartbeat. Lub is low-pitched, long, and occurs during **systole**, when the ventricles contract and the mitral and tricuspid valves between the atria and ventricles close. Dub is a sharp snap heard during **diastole**, when the ventricles relax and the semilunar valves in the pulmonary artery and aortic artery close. Diastole takes more time than systole, so there is a brief pause after the dub before the next lub when the heart is beating normally. **Extra sounds can indicate fluid overload.** A **cardiac friction rub** may be heard in a uremic or underdialyzed patient, which is a symptom of **pericarditis** (inflammation of the sac surrounding the heart). Complete absence of heart sounds can be due to a patient with a very thick chest wall or to life-threatening cardiac tamponade. If any abnormalities are heard in heart sounds, report them to nurse immediately.

PULSE

The patient's pulse should be measured prior to dialysis and compared against the following rates:

- Normal Rates:
  - Adult at rest: 60-100 bpm
  - Child <12: 80-100 bpm
  - Toddler: >100 bpm
  - Infant <1 year: 100-140 bpm
  - Newborn (neonate): 150 bpm
  - Very fit athletes: 45-60 bpm

- Abnormal Rates:
  - o Bradycardia (slow heart rate): <50 bpm
  - o Tachycardia (fast heart rate): >100 bpm

Check pulse and respirations simultaneously, so the patient does not subconsciously alter their breathing rate. Do not check with the thumb, as one's own pulse may be felt; use fingertips. Chart the rate, rhythm, and quality of the patient's pulse.

APICAL PULSE

To find the patient's apical pulse, count to the 5th rib space in the middle of the left side of the chest or midclavicular line. If the apical pulse is regular, count for 30 seconds, multiply it by two, and record the reading. If the apical pulse is irregular, count for a full minute and record the reading. Report an irregular pulse to the nurse to evaluate for a possible pulse deficit. A **pulse deficit** occurs when the radial pulse in the wrist is slower than the apical pulse in the chest. A pulse deficit can indicate the patient has weak heart contractions, which fail to transmit beats to the arterial system. To properly assess the dialysis patient for pulse deficit, the nurse and an assistant should count the apical and radial pulses at the same time and compare the result.

TEMPERATURE

When recording oral temperature, the purpose is to help the nurse evaluate complications occurring before, during, or after treatment. Temperature should be taken and recorded both pre-dialysis and post-dialysis. The hemodialysis technician should be familiar with the following **values and ranges as they pertain to body temperature**:

- Ideal body temperature 98.6 °F (37 °C); Normal range 97.8 °F (36.5 °C) - 99 °F (37.2 °C)
- Patients with kidney disease tend to have a lower oral temperature (~96.8 °F or 36 °C)
- Hypothermia <95 °F (<35 °C)
- Pyrexia (fever) >99 °F (37 °C) oral or >99.8 °F rectal (37.6 °C)
- Hyperpyrexia 107.6 °F (>42 °C)
- Critical value: Report any oral temperature elevation over 100 °F (37.7 °C) to the nurse, who then verifies the oral reading with a more accurate rectal or arterial temperature.

Significance:

- Establishes the patient's baseline.
- Elevations from baseline before dialysis indicate infection or ovulation.
- Elevation from baseline after dialysis starts indicate progeny reaction/high dialysate temperature.
- Hypothermia can result from uremia, sepsis, diabetes, Addison's disease, liver failure, hypothyroidism, hypothalamus problems, street drugs/alcohol, lithium, barbiturates, opiates, benzodiazepines, phenothiazines, or clonidine.

Patient Instructions:

- No smoking, eating, or drinking for 30 minutes prior to the reading.
- Refrain from talking during an oral reading, as it lowers the temperature.

BREATH SOUNDS AND RESPIRATIONS

The hemodialysis technician should be aware of the following with regards to assessing respirations and breath sounds:

- **Normal rates**: Adults: 12-20 bpm, Children <12: 20-30 bpm, Newborns: 30-60 bpm; Rate increases with exercise or emotions and can be consciously controlled.
- **Normal sounds**: Clear, audible sounds heard completely to bases of both lungs. Even rhythm, except for an occasional deep breath.

The hemodialysis technician must alert the nurse of any of the following:

- Diminished sounds.
- **Crackles (rales)**: Discontinuous sound like hair rubbed between fingers, heard during inspiration in pulmonary edema and early-stage pneumonia. Ask the patient to cough.
  - **Coarse crackles** are low-pitched and sound wet.
  - **Fine crackles** are high-pitched and sound dry.
- **Dyspnea**: Difficult breathing.
- **Orthopnea**: Inability to breathe (or difficulty breathing) while lying down.
- **Pleural friction rub**: Low-pitched grating sound similar to leather rubbing against leather heard during inhalation in pleurisy.
- **Rhonchi**: Low-pitched, snoring, rumbling sounds heard continuously during expiration, indicating mucus congestion or bronchitis.
- **Shortness of breath**: Can indicate fluid in the lungs from fluid overload.
- **Stridor**: High-pitched crowing during inspiration that occurs when the larynx or trachea is narrowed or obstructed by a foreign object, airway damage, allergy, croup, acute laryngitis, or enlarged tonsils. Stridor is a medical emergency, especially in a child.
- **Wheezing**: High-pitched whistling from air pushed through narrowed passages. Louder during expiration. Most often heard in emphysema, asthma, and anaphylaxis.

> **Review Video: Lung Sounds**
> Visit mometrix.com/academy and enter code: 765616

PATIENT WEIGHT

Keeping track of patient weight and weight changes is an important part of patient care, because weight and weight changes are used to determine the efficacy of the dialysis treatment. Dialysis patients are weighed before and after a dialysis treatment. This is called the pre-dialysis weight and the post-dialysis weight. Pre-dialysis weight can be used to determine the level of ultrafiltration that the patient requires. Post-dialysis weight demonstrates the level of ultrafiltration that took place during the hemodialysis treatment. Patients may keep track of their weight on a regular basis to determine if their fluid intake is appropriate. Weight can be used to assess fluid balance control between dialysis treatments. A weight gain occurring between dialysis treatments indicates fluid retention. The patient is usually encouraged to restrict weight gain to 1 pound per day.

PROCEDURE FOR COLLECTING PATIENT WEIGHT PRIOR TO DIALYSIS

When weighing the patient before dialysis, the patient should be weighted on the same scales and wearing the same amount of clothing for each session. Compare the current reading to both the patient's last pre-dialysis weight and post-dialysis weight. Subtract the last session's post-weight from the current pre-weight to determine the amount of gain between treatments. The recommended weight gain between treatments is usually in the range of 3.5-4.5 lb. The last post-treatment weight may not necessarily be the patient's prescribed dry weight. Look at the last several treatment logs to see if the patient is achieving the prescribed dry weight. Ask the patient if he/she feels abdominal or limb cramping, or dizziness from hypotension. If so, contact the nurse.

DRY WEIGHT

The patient's **dry weight** is the weight at which he/she is free of any excess fluid. Dry weight changes over time, as the patient gains or loses muscle weight. A patient who has achieved dry weight has:

- No edema present.
- Clear breath sounds bilaterally.
- Blood pressure (BP) within normal limits for the individual.

There is no exact formula for determining dry weight; it is a combination of the careful assessment of several factors. The patient at ideal dry weight should not be accompanied by hypotension, dizziness, or cramping during treatment. If these events occur, consult the nurse about raising the dry or target weight. If the patient is leaving treatment with edema, hypertension, or lung congestion, consult the nurse about lowering the dry or target weight.

ASSESSING FOR PHYSICAL ISSUES AND EDEMA

The patient is assessed prior to receiving every dialysis treatment. The hemodialysis technician should ask the patient about his or her health. The patient should be asked if he or she has been experiencing any health problems, such as headaches or diarrhea. The hemodialysis technician should take note of the patient's demeanor, speech, and mentation prior to treatment.

Fluid may accumulate in abnormal amounts in the body tissues. This is called **edema**. If the patient gains an excessive amount of weight between dialysis treatments, edema may result. Different parts of the body may be affected by edema. The patient may exhibit swelling in the ankle, sacrum, or face. Fluid overload may also result in distension of the jugular veins. Before a dialysis treatment, the patient is assessed for accumulated fluid. The level of ultrafiltration is based on the amount of accumulated fluid.

APPEARANCE AND SIGNIFICANCE OF PERIPHERAL EDEMA

Edema occurs from **hypo-albuminemia** (>3 grams protein lost per day) with **salt and water retention.** This state is common in patients with end-stage renal disease (ESRD/ dropsy), cirrhosis of the liver (ascites), congestive heart failure (CHF), anaphylaxis, hypothyroidism, varicose veins, deep vein thrombosis, preeclampsia, safety valve lymphatic insufficiency, beriberi, protein malnutrition (kwashiorkor), celiac disease, or filariasis (elephantiasis). Signs of edema in the ambulatory patient include swollen hands, feet, face, eyelids; distended abdomen; and/or bulging neck veins. Look for swelling of the hips and sacrum in a bed-bound patient. Press the swelling with the thumb for 5 seconds to record the level of edema.

Result	Write	Pronounce
Barely discernable indentation (2 mm); rebounds immediately	+1 edema	One plus or mild pitting edema
3-4 mm indentation; rebounds in <15 sec	+2 edema	Two plus or moderate pitting edema
5-6 mm indentation; rebounds in 10-30 sec	+3 edema	Three plus or moderate to severe pitting edema

| >7 mm indentation; rebounds in >20 sec | +4 edema | Four plus or severe pitting edema |
| Severe, widespread edema in all tissues & cavities simultaneously | Anasarca | |

ASSESSING FOR JUGULAR VEIN DISTENTION

To evaluate for jugular vein distention, first place the patient in supine rest position (on the back, facing up). Elevate the head of the bed 30-45°. The patient's head and neck should be in a neutral position, without flexion. The jugular veins in the neck become readily visible. Note the highest visible point of the jugular veins, measured from the suprasternal notch. Ask the patient to sit up. Normally, jugular veins flatten out when a person sits up. When the jugular veins are distended in a sitting position, this may indicate heart disease or fluid overload. Bilateral elevations over 3 cm are considered abnormal. Chart findings and notify the nurse of any abnormalities.

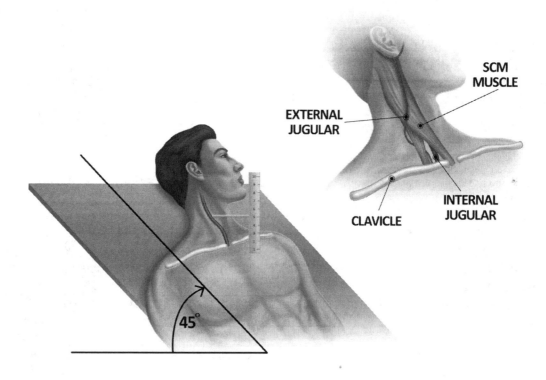

ASSESSING FOR INFECTION

SIGNS AND SYMPTOMS OF ACCESS INFECTION

A sign is an objective problem that can be observed by the hemodialysis technician. A symptom is a subjective problem that the patient self-reports. **Signs and symptoms of infection** in an access include pain, fever, redness, warmth over the graft, swelling, and drainage at the access site. Infections can also occur without any obvious symptoms because patients with ESRD are immunosuppressed. Observe fistulas and AV grafts for open areas (skin breakdown). Central venous catheters are particularly susceptible to infection and can lead to sepsis (blood poisoning), a life-threatening condition that requires removal of the catheter and treatment with antibiotics. Report any suspected symptoms of access infection to the nurse in charge of the patient. Collect blood cultures and swabs per order. Prompt treatment of access infections helps to preserve the life of the access.

35

SIGNS OF SYSTEMIC INFECTION

Always question the patient at the beginning of each treatment about possible signs and symptoms of generalized infection. Patients with renal disease have altered immune function and are more susceptible to infection than the general population (**immunosuppression**). Infections in this population happen more frequently and are more severe. These patients with severe infections may lack the normal fever response seen in other populations. Patients with diabetes and renal disease heal very slowly. Patients with central line access are frequently prone to infection. Check all accesses at each treatment for the presence of redness, warmth, swelling, or drainage. Urinary tract infections are another major cause of infection in patients with renal disease and clinical symptoms, such as pain and cloudy or odorous urine, may be absent. These patients frequently have **anuria** (absence of urine) or **oliguria** (abnormally scanty urine), so the nurse may obtain a urine sample for culture, chemistry, and cytology by catheterizing the patient.

SIGNS AND SYMPTOMS OF ACCESS STENOSIS

Stenosis is a narrowing or occlusion of the internal lumen of a vascular access. Blood backwashes near the stenosed area and can lead to clotting of the access. A decrease in thrill along the course of a graft may indicate stenosis or an impending clot. A change in the sound of the bruit may also indicate stenosis. Stenosis of the access leads to increased pressure within the vessel and may cause prolonged bleeding of the puncture sites after needles are removed. If a 16-gauge needle is used with a blood flow pressure of 200 mL/min, then venous pressures should be less than 150 mmHg. If a 15-gauge needle is used, the venous pressure should be less than 100 mmHg.

ASSESSING FOR HEMOSTASIS AND ORTHOSTATIC HYPOTENSION

Additional pre-dialysis assessment includes the following:

- **Hemostasis**: Laboratory findings, such as skin bleeding time, platelet count, fibrinogen, thrombin time (TT), prothrombin time (PT), and partial thromboplastin time (aPTT) should be evaluated to help predict the risk of bleeding. Additionally, the patient should be assessed for signs of bleeding (bruising, petechiae, bleeding gums, and blood in the urine if producing urine).
- **Orthostatic hypotension**: The patient's blood pressure should be taken in standing and sitting position prior to dialysis and checked approximately every 30 minutes during treatment. At the conclusion of treatment, a sitting blood pressure should be taken followed by a standing blood pressure to determine if the patient is experiencing a pronounced drop in blood pressure. Orthostatic hypotension is usually defined as a drop in systolic blood pressure of 20 mmHg and drop in diastolic pressure of 10 mmHg. Some drop in blood pressure is common when a person stands, but this should rapidly stabilize (check every 3 minutes).

ASSESSING FOR THE NEED FOR SUPPLEMENTAL OXYGEN

Patients may require supplemental oxygen during hemodialysis, especially patients with a history of heart diseases or venous oxygen saturation of less than 60%. Blood oxygen levels decrease during hemodialysis by up to 23%, and the patient may experience signs of hypoxia, such as muscle cramping, light-headedness, blurred vision, confusion, nausea, shortness of breath, and tissue hypoxia as a result. Oxygen saturation should be assessed prior to beginning dialysis. In addition to patients with underlying heart disease, oxygen should be administered to patients who appear in respiratory distress and those whose SpO_2 falls below 94% during treatment (<90% is clinically significant). Because patients often fall asleep during treatment, those with sleep apnea should also receive supplemental oxygen. Blood oxygenation may be assessed through pulse oximetry, blood gas analysis, or use of a blood volume monitor on the arterial end of the dialyzer. The goal of oxygen therapy is to maintain the oxygen saturation at 94-98%.

EIGHT FINAL CHECKS PRIOR TO DIALYSIS

The final eight checks that must be done before placing a patient on dialysis include:

- Recheck the physician's orders to ensure that the correct dialyzer is being used.
- If using a reprocessed dialyzer, verify the name on the dialyzer is correct and check the dialyzer for residual sterilant (bleach and formaldehyde).
- Verify that the correct dialysate concentrate is being used.
- Ensure that the blood circuit is primed with saline.
- Recheck all line connections for security and kinks.
- Check all machine alarms to ensure they are functioning normally.
- Verify that the pre-dialysis assessment has been completed.
- Double check the patient's access to ensure that needles or catheter connections are secure.

These eight steps are absolutely necessary for providing the patient with quality treatment.

Evaluate, Intervene, and Manage Treatment: Pre-Treatment

DIALYSIS ADEQUACY

Dialysis adequacy is determined by Kt/V (total urea removal per volume) and URR (urea reduction ratio). These measures are used to assess how well the dialysis is working. Dialysis is considered optimal if it allows the patient to live a healthy life for almost as many years as he or she would have lived if the patient did not have end-stage renal disease. Guidelines to determine acceptable dialysis adequacy have been established by the National Kidney Foundation. Individual dialysis clinics may set their own, more stringent goals. Higher delivered doses of dialysis are associated with better outcomes for the patient. Dialysis adequacy is used to determine the dialysis prescription. If the dialysis is not adequate, the patient's health will suffer.

KT/V

The object of dialysis treatment is to remove waste products from the body. Kt/V is a measure of the adequacy of dialysis treatment. Kt/V is a ratio. K stands for dialyzer clearance of urea, and t stands for dialysis time. V stands for the volume of distribution of urea in the patient's body fluid. Therefore, Kt/V is the ratio of the dialyzer clearance of urea multiplied by the dialysis time in relationship to the total body water. The Kidney Disease Outcomes Quality Initiative clinical practice guidelines recommend that delivered Kt/V should be at least 1.2.

URR

URR is the abbreviation for **urea reduction ratio**. It is used to assess the effectiveness of hemodialysis treatment. URR is based on levels of urea (BUN or blood urea nitrogen) in the blood. The test involves the measurement of the BUN before and after dialysis treatment. In this way, it measures the amount that the blood urea has decreased after dialysis. URR is a reflection of the dose of dialysis delivered. The Kidney Disease Outcomes Quality Initiative clinical practice guidelines no longer recommend that URR be used as the primary measurement of dialysis adequacy due to issues with precision, while other experts recommend a URR of at least 65%. A lower URR value is suggestive of a shorter survival time for dialysis patients. The URR may be used with Kt/V, or on its own. Different centers use one or both tests.

INFLUENCING FACTORS

The effectiveness of dialysis can be adversely affected by a number of factors. Urea clearance can be impeded by access recirculation, a less than adequate flow of blood from vascular access, inadequate reprocessing by the dialyzer, dialyzer fibers that are clotted, improperly calibrated equipment, inappropriate flow rates of blood and dialysate, dialyzer leaks, and equipment malfunctions. An inadequate treatment time may result from the premature termination of a particular treatment, and miscalculation in timing. Laboratory or testing errors can cause dialysis to be less than optimal in a number of ways:

- The BUN sample may be diluted with saline.
- The pre-dialysis BUN sample may be drawn after the dialysis has been started.
- The post-dialysis BUN may be drawn before the dialysis treatment has ended.
- The BUN may be drawn more than 5 minutes after the dialysis treatment has ended.

UREA KINETIC MODELING

Urea kinetic modeling (UKM) is used to monitor the effects of dialysis and to assess the protein intake of a dialysis patient. A definitive method for conducting UKM has not been established. Its use, however, is standard practice in facilities that conduct hemodialysis and peritoneal dialysis. UKM requires the use of a computer due to the complex mathematical calculations involved. BUN levels before and after a particular dialysis treatment are entered into a computer database. If the patient is still urinating, residual urea clearance is also entered. Details about the patient and his or her dialysis treatment are also a part of the calculation. These details include the age, weight, sex, and hematocrit of the patient. In addition, the rate of blood flow, rate of dialysate flow, dialyzer clearance data, the length of the specific treatment, and the interdialytic interval are included.

BLOOD FLOW RATE

Most blood pumps feature speed indicators to gauge the flow rate of blood. The speed indicator and the internal diameter of the tubing must match, or the indicator will not produce accurate results regarding speed of blood flow. The speed indicator of the pump should be checked regularly. To check the calibration of the speed indicator, the same brand and lot of tubing should be used. To check the rate of flow, water of 37 °C is pumped through the tubing. The tubing is partially clamped to simulate the negative pressure that occurs during a dialysis treatment. The test should be run for 3-5 minutes and a graduated cylinder should be used to catch the outflow. The flow rate is calculated by dividing the volume (mL) by time (min).

SETTING THE DIALYSIS FLOW RATE AND ITS IMPACT ON ADEQUACY

The blood flow rate for hemodialysis is generally 300-500 mL/min (average 400 in the United States), but the rate for the individual patient may depend on the size and maturity of the access as well as the needle size. With initiation, the blood flow rate is set low and raised slowly to tolerance. Higher flow rates (>400 mL/min) are more effective at removing toxins, such as urea. The flow rate for dialysate (which typically flows in the opposite direction as the blood flow) is usually 500-800 mL/min. Higher dialysate flow rates more effectively remove urea from the blood. However, higher blood flow rates may result in increased trauma to the vessels and hemolysis. The flow rate depends to some degree on the type of hemodialysis machine, with conventional machines requiring a blood flow rate to dialysate flow rate ratio of 1:2 but other systems (such as NxStage) requiring a ratio of 1:3.

DIALYSATE SOLUTION PRESCRIPTION

Dialysate solution is prescribed by a doctor, who individualizes it to the patient's needs. Double check to ensure the machine has been connected to the correct dialysate before starting dialysis treatment. Solutions are available with different concentrations of potassium and calcium, or no potassium. Also, some machines allow different sodium profiles or models, with sodium starting at higher concentrations at the beginning of treatment and tapering off toward the end of treatment. Ensure that the correct sodium model for the patient is being used if one is ordered; never change it without a physician's order, or substitute another type. As sodium levels in the blood rise, so do potassium levels. If the patient enters treatment already in a hyperkalemic state (serum potassium level >5 mmol/L), administering high salt dialysate increases irritability of the central nervous system and cardiac conduction pathways, causing weakness and hyporeflexia. Hyperkalemia treatment includes IV calcium, bicarbonate, glucose, and insulin; albuterol and epinephrine; cation-exchange resins; and changes in diet, diuretics, and dialysis treatment.

INSPECTING THE DIALYZER

The first duty of the hemodialysis technician is to ensure that the patient receives a safe and effective dialysis treatment. Inattention in a dialysis unit has harmful or fatal consequences. High blood pump speeds without proper connections can quickly drain a patient's full blood volume onto the floor, a chair, or bed. The patient's blood volume is about 5 liters. **Should a line connection separate**, it takes as little as 10 minutes for full blood loss to occur at a 500 mL/min blood flow rate. Ensure all tubing connections are secure. Only after completing the eight final checks should the arterial line be unclamped and the blood pump turned on. Release the venous line clamp gently and slowly, to prevent a rush of pressure from causing the access to infiltrate. If wasting the prime, the venous end of the tubing remains over a receptacle until the blood reaches the venous drip chamber. Never leave a patient's chair—even for a moment—until the blood pump reaches full speed and his/her first set of vital signs have been taken and recorded.

TEMPORARY VASCULAR ACCESS

Temporary vascular access using a central venous catheter (CVC) is sometimes used in hemodialysis. A catheter may be used for access in a case of acute dialysis. A catheter may also be used to dialyze a patient if a kidney transplant is imminent. A catheter is sometimes used while the arteriovenous fistula is maturing. If an internal access is not possible because of a lack of suitable vessels, a catheter may be used as a permanent access. If the patient is undergoing plasmapheresis, a catheter may be used for hemodialysis. A catheter is used with patients receiving venovenous continuous renal replacement therapy. A catheter may be used on a temporary basis for patients receiving peritoneal dialysis. This may be necessary if the patient develops peritonitis.

VEINS USED FOR TEMPORARY ACCESS

The catheter for temporary access may be inserted into the **jugular vein** (pictured below), the **femoral vein,** the **subclavian vein,** or in rare circumstances, the **lumbar vein.** The National Kidney Foundation makes the recommendation of considering temporary access locations in the following order of priority: internal jugular vein, external jugular vein, femoral vein, subclavian vein, and lumbar vein. The catheter has two lumens to permit two-way blood flow. Subclavian catheters and jugular catheters should not be used in all patients. The subclavian and jugular vein catheters are inserted while the patient is in the supine or Trendelenburg position. If the patient cannot be placed in the supine position or in the Trendelenburg position due to respiratory problems, the subclavian and jugular catheters are contraindicated. If the patient has subclavian vein stenosis, subclavian and jugular catheters are contraindicated. If the catheter will be needed for longer than 3 weeks, it is tunneled under the skin. This is more comfortable for the patient and reduces complications.

SUBCLAVIAN AND JUGULAR VEIN CATHETER INSERTION

The insertion of the subclavian or jugular catheter requires the use of aseptic technique. The patient is placed in the supine or Trendelenburg position. The head is turned to the side opposite the surgical site. The area around the surgical site is cleaned using normal surgical technique and draped. The catheter is inserted after the administration of a local anesthetic. The catheter is sutured to ensure that it stays in place. The correct placement of the catheter must be verified before it can be used. The complications of surgery to insert a subclavian or jugular catheter include the following: pneumothorax, hemothorax, air embolism, and severe bleeding. Severe bleeding may occur if an artery is punctured during the procedure.

FEMORAL CATHETER INSERTION

A femoral catheter is a type of temporary access and is used under certain conditions. A femoral catheter is often used when a jugular catheter is contraindicated. A femoral catheter may be inserted when the patient is confined to bed, when the patient has end-stage renal disease and a blocked internal access, when continuous renal replacement therapy is necessary, and in the case of a patient with subclavian renal stenosis. There are possible complications involved with the insertion of a femoral catheter. If the vein is punctured during insertion of the catheter, a retroperitoneal hemorrhage can occur. In addition, there may be severe bleeding at the site of insertion. The femoral site is at higher risk for infections due to its location on the body.

TUNNELED CATHETER

A tunneled catheter is threaded through the internal jugular vein or the subclavian vein (pictured below). The catheter is inserted into the wall of the chest and exits the body approximately six inches from the site of insertion. The tunneled catheter becomes fixed in place. The tunneled catheter is used if the patient requires multiple treatments each day for a prolonged period of time, typically more than 3 months, but National Kidney Foundation guidelines recommend transitioning to an AV graft or fistula if able to do so for patients requiring chronic long-term dialysis. Infection occurs commonly in individuals with tunneled catheters (though infection risk is less in tunneled catheters than non-tunneled catheters). These catheters must be monitored closely because of the risk of infection, and 10-15% of the time the catheter must be removed because an infection has developed. A permanent catheter may also be inserted into the mammary veins or the femoral vein.

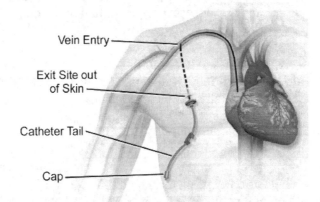

Tunneled Central Venous Access Device

CARING FOR THE PATIENT WITH A CENTRAL VENOUS CATHETER

Central venous catheters provide temporary access when the patient has acute kidney failure and is awaiting a graft or fistula, or requires emergency hemodialysis. Use aseptic technique at all times when dialyzing the patient with a central venous catheter, because he/she is highly prone to sepsis, local infection, and stenosis. The tip of a central venous catheter is in very close proximity to the heart via the superior vena cava. Place sterile drapes or 4" × 4" gauze pads under the catheter hubs to provide a germ-free field. Wrap the caps and hubs with sterile gauze soaked in a disinfectant per unit policy at the beginning and ending of treatment. Perform exit site care aseptically, using a disinfectant appropriate for the type of catheter, working from the exit site outward in a spiral motion. Apply a sterile dressing. Report signs and symptoms of infection, such as redness or drainage, to the nurse immediately.

PERMANENT VASCULAR ACCESS

A permanent vascular access has to be established in patients requiring chronic hemodialysis. The National Kidney Foundation has set guidelines for selecting vascular access. The guidelines recommend that a native arteriovenous (AV) fistula serve as the permanent access for the majority of chronic hemodialysis patients due to lower incidence of complications when compared to an AV graft. AV fistulae and AV grafts are preferred to a permanent CVC. Permanent access sites include the following: wrist primary arteriovenous fistula, elbow primary arteriovenous fistula, arteriovenous graft of synthetic material, transposed brachiobasilic vein fistula, and cuffed tunneled central venous catheter.

ARTERIOVENOUS FISTULA (AV FISTULA)

An AV fistula is a surgically created internal access used for hemodialysis. This type of access uses the patient's blood vessels to create access for the dialysis treatment. The surgeon creating an internal arteriovenous fistula makes a 5-mm opening in an adjacent vein and artery. The vein and artery are joined at this point forming the AV fistula. The artery and vein are connected by anastomosis side to side, end to end, or end to side. The vein becomes enlarged due to the extra blood entering it from the artery. This enlargement of the vein permits large gauge needles to be positioned for dialysis. The access resulting from the formation of the fistula will produce a flow of blood in the range of 300-500 mL/min.

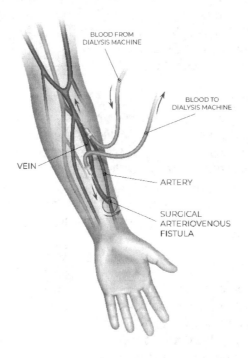

PLACEMENT

An arteriovenous fistula can be established in the **upper or lower arm**. The radial artery and cephalic vein of the lower arm and the brachial artery and cephalic vein of the upper arm are often used to create an arteriovenous fistula. The choice of access site depends on the patient's vasculature. The selection of vessels that are less than optimal for the purpose can result in failure of the arteriovenous fistula. The access site can be chosen with the use of venography. Venography can help rule out unsuitable sites. Doppler flow studies can also be used to pick a suitable site for the fistula. If at all possible, the arteriovenous fistula is established in the patient's nondominant hand to lessen the effects of the fistula on the patient's daily activities. This also allows the patient to self-cannulate if necessary.

CANNULATION

A new AV fistula must be treated with care during **cannulation**. Before maturation, the fistula is fragile. At first, only one needle may be inserted into the AV fistula. This is the arterial outflow. In this case, the venous return occurs through the central venous catheter. For the first cannulations, a smaller-gauge needle may be used with lower rates of blood flow.

The long-term patency of the access depends on the **placement of the arterial and venous needles**. Placing the needles in the same spot during each treatment will lead to thinning of the walls of the vessels and aneurysms. Therefore, this practice should be avoided. The needles should not be inserted in sites of weakness in the walls of the vessels. From treatment to treatment, the entire length of the access should be utilized for insertion.

HASTENING ENLARGEMENT OF VEINS

The fistula must be allowed to heal for 4-5 days before any attempt is made to hasten the speed of **vein enlargement**. After this time, a tourniquet or pressure cuff may be used to increase the speed of vein enlargement. The device is tied snugly around the upper arm, left in position for half an hour, and removed. This process may be repeated a number of times each day. Used in this way the tourniquet or pressure cuff will cause the distention of the veins. Squeezing a rubber ball while the tourniquet is in position may also help to speed up the enlargement of the vein. Warm compresses may also facilitate this process.

ARTERIOVENOUS GRAFT (AV GRAFT)

An AV graft is used when a native AV fistula cannot be created due to inadequate vessels. An AV graft is usually made of synthetic material, but biologic material can be used. The AV graft material is surgically implanted under the skin in the upper or lower arm. If the AV graft cannot be implanted in the arm. the graft may be implanted in the chest or leg. The AV graft involves bridging the artery and vein with the graft material. The graft may be configured in a number of ways. It may be straight, looped, or curved. The graft causes the blood to flow from the artery to the vein. The graft can be used to provide access 2-6 weeks after surgical implantation. The cannulation needles are inserted into the graft material.

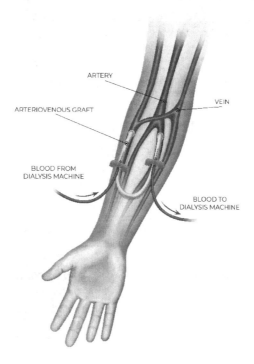

DIRECTION OF BLOOD FLOW

The blood flows from the artery to the vein. The venous needle should be positioned with the blood flow. If the needle is incorrectly placed so that it goes against the blood flow, it will create increased resistance to the blood leaving the dialyzer as it returns to the patient.

Depressing the AV graft at midpoint will block the flow of blood. A bruit can be listened for, or a thrill can be felt for, on either side of the occlusion. The blood will still be entering the arterial side, and a bruit will be heard and or a thrill felt. The blood will be prevented from entering the venous side, and little or no bruit will be heard and no thrill felt. The flow can also be determined once the needles have been positioned. When the graft is compressed at midpoint, a flashback of blood will occur in the arterial needle.

BASILIC VEIN TRANSPOSITION

Basilic vein transposition is a method used to create access for dialysis in a patient with unsuitable arteries and veins in the wrist. The technique involves the transposition of vessels. The basilic vein is dissected and transposed anteriorly and subcutaneously. An anastomosis is then formed between the basilic vein and the brachial artery. This surgical procedure permits cannulation by creating a large surface area. The surgery requires a large incision, running from the mid-antecubital fossa up the medical surface of the arm and ending at the axilla. This procedure allows the surgeon to avoid using a synthetic graft, which has a higher risk of infection.

VASCULAR ACCESS IN PEDIATRIC PATIENTS

It is more difficult to establish vascular access in pediatric patients. In the case of patients weighing less than 10 kg, access must be established using a catheter placed in a major vessel. Catheters come in different sizes, and a catheter of appropriate size must be used. The catheter must not be so big that it blocks normal blood flow in the vein. Patients weighing more than 10 kg may be candidates for an arteriovenous loop graft positioned in the thigh. Patients weighing more than 15 kg may be candidates for a primary arteriovenous fistula positioned in the forearm. If the patient weighs less than 20 kg, creation of a permanent access is very difficult and should only be attempted by an experienced surgeon or pediatric nephrologist.

ASSESSING ACCESS

VISUALLY INSPECTING THE GRAFT OR FISTULA PRIOR TO DIALYSIS

Carefully observe the graft or fistula before each dialysis session for the following:

Infection:

- Fever (not always present in immunosuppressed patients)
- Redness (erythema)
- Warmth over the graft
- Swelling (edema)
- Drainage
- Open sores
- Abscesses (pimples near scabs of previous needle insertions, which are actually large, pus-filled cavities below the skin)

Aneurysm:

- A weak, thinned, bulging area in the access

Pseudoaneurysm:

- Hematoma (hard blood tumor under the skin)
- Fibrous tissue continues to enlarge
- Murmurs
- Pulsation

Assessing Access Patency

Every fistula or graft should have a strong pulse, called a **thrill**. The hemodialysis technician should be able to feel the thrill by lightly palpating along the entire length of the access. Be careful not to compress the graft or fistula during palpation, as this can occlude the access and obliterate the pulse. The thrill should feel like a pounding or buzzing with each heartbeat. Some patients describe it as feeling like the buzz of electricity.

After finding the thrill, also listen over the entire length of the access with a stethoscope for a strong, steady swooshing sound, called a **bruit**. If the hemodialysis technician notes any changes in the sound along the length, they should bring them to the attention of the nurse for assessment. Absence of a thrill or bruit may mean that the access has clotted. The doctor may be able to remove the clot (**thrombectomy**) through a percutaneous balloon-assisted aspiration in the Radiology Department.

Assessing Catheter Patency

Verify **catheter patency** by pulling back on each limb of the catheter with a syringe to remove the 3-5 mL of standing heparin that is used to prevent the ports from clotting between treatments. Always pull back on the syringe until blood is visualized. This ensures that all the heparin is removed and the patient will not receive more than is ordered during dialysis. After aspirating, flush each port with 10 mL of sterile normal saline. It should be easy to aspirate and flush both limbs of the catheter. If any resistance is met, notify the nurse in charge of the patient. The patient may have developed access stenosis.

Palpating Blood Flow Direction in a Fistula and Graft

Palpation is an important assessment technique because it affects how to place the needles and the resulting effectiveness of the patient's dialysis:

- To find the direction of blood flow in a **fistula**, feel for a bump near the incision line. The strongest pulse should be felt over this bump. Partially occlude the fistula at the middle point by pressing on it. Feel the pulse on both sides of the occluded portion. The side with the strongest pulse is the arterial side. The blood flow in a fistula will always be from the anastomosis through the veins and back to the heart.
- To find the direction of blood flow in a **graft**, compress the middle portion of the graft and feel each side for a pulse. The side with the strongest pulse is the arterial portion of the graft.

Two other techniques are **auscultation** (listening to the pulse with a stethoscope), and **sticking the graft and observing the flashback**. The side with the strongest flashback is the arterial side.

Assessing Internal Access

The internal access should be assessed before cleaning or cannulation. The access should first be observed visually for signs of infection. The temperature of the skin at the access should be normal. Heat is often an indication of infection and a cool site may indicate thrombosis. The previous needle insertion sites should be checked to ensure proper healing. The skin at the access should be of normal color and without signs of bruising. Swelling may be visible due to poor venous drainage or because of a previous needle insertion. Swelling of the site should be monitored to determine if the condition is improving or deteriorating. The site should be checked to ensure that circulation is adequate and that the access is patent. The internal access should be palpated to determine if there is an appropriate thrill through the length of the vessel.

CANNULATION

POSITIONING OF HEMODIALYSIS NEEDLES

Blood flow may be described as antegrade or retrograde. Antegrade is a term referring to movement in the direction of the flow of blood, and retrograde means movement against the flow of blood. The **venous needle must be placed in an antegrade position**. This is toward the heart. The **arterial needle may be placed in an antegrade or retrograde position.** In other words, it may be placed toward the heart or toward the hand. The arterial needle is the one placed nearer to the anastomosis, but it must be placed at least 3 mm away. The position of the venous needle must be placed a minimum of 5 cm proximal to the arterial needle.

ASEPTIC TECHNIQUE AND NEEDLE TYPES FOR AV FISTULA ACCESS

Before cannulation, an **antiseptic** solution should be used on the skin around the fistula. A solution such as chlorhexidine gluconate or povidone-iodine may be used. The antiseptic solution should be applied in a circular motion from the puncture site outward. An area of 2 inches in diameter should be cleaned. Before the needle is inserted, the antiseptic solution must be permitted to dry on the skin.

The preferred needles for use with an AV fistula are large-gauge, thin wall, back-eye needles. High-flux and high-efficiency dialysis require larger gauge needles. Large, 14-gauge needles may permit blood flows of 400-500 mL/min. Smaller needles (17-gauge) are used with children and infants. For a blood flow of 350 mL/min or greater, a 15-gauge needle is recommended. If a high blood flow rate is required, using a small gauge needle may result in hemolysis of the red blood cells.

BUTTONHOLE TECHNIQUE

The buttonhole technique is also called the constant-site technique. This technique has been used to cannulate arteriovenous fistulas for approximately 25 years. This technique involves the repeated insertion of the needle at the same angle and in the same spot. This method creates a permanent tunnel of scar tissue called a buttonhole. The needle is inserted through this tunnel with each cannulation. This method is less painful for the patient and there are fewer incidents of infiltration than occur with other methods. This is a useful technique for patients who use an at-home dialyzer. A buttonhole needle set with anti-stick dull bevels is available for use with an established buttonhole. The anti-stick dull bevel prevents the tissue around the scar tissue from being sliced during insertion.

USE OF ANESTHETIC

The insertion of a needle into the dialysis access may cause pain or discomfort. This is especially true when the patient has a new access. **Intradermal anesthetic** may be administered to ease the discomfort. An anesthetic, such as lidocaine 1% (Xylocaine), can be used for this purpose. The anesthetic is injected just under the top of the skin. The needle is inserted at a 15-degree angle. The individual administering the anesthetic must be sure to aspirate before injection to ensure that the needle is not in a blood vessel. If blood is withdrawn during aspiration, the syringe must be discarded. A topical anesthetic, such as EMLA cream, may also be applied to prevent discomfort during needle insertion. The topical anesthetic is applied before the patient arrives for treatment, and removed before cannulation.

EQUIPMENT AND PROCEDURE FOR THE ADMINISTRATION OF LIDOCAINE

Equipment:

- 1% lidocaine
- Chlorhexidine skin cleanser

- 1 cc or tuberculin syringe
- Sterile gauze

Procedure:

1. Examine fistula or graft to ensure it is a good site for needles (thrill, bruit, intact skin, no signs of infection).
2. Cleanse skin over insertion site with chlorhexidine swab in a spiral pattern, from inside to outside.
3. Allow site to air dry; avoid touching cleansed skin.
4. Aspirate lidocaine into a 1 cc or tuberculin syringe for each site; tap out air bubbles.
5. Insert cannula tip just under skin's surface—some grafts and fistulae are very superficial.
6. Pull back slightly on plunger. Ensure no blood enters syringe.
7. Inject enough lidocaine to form a small wheal. Lidocaine burns, so use only a little bit. Do not inject lidocaine directly into graft.
8. Remove syringe and quickly cover wheal with sterile gauze to absorb any leaking lidocaine or blood drops.

ACCESS CARE
FISTULA CARE

A fistula requires care. In the case of a new fistula, the arm should be elevated and placed on a soft surface. This will help prevent the arm from swelling. After the needle has been removed following any hemodialysis treatment, pressure must be kept on the puncture sites for 10-20 minutes. The source of the pressure can be the hand or a pressure dressing. The heparin used during treatment can cause serious bleeding from the fistula. Bleeding under the skin can cause the formation of a hematoma and can also cause the formation of scar tissue. If the bleeding after hemodialysis is too severe or continues for longer than 20 minutes after the needles have been removed from the fistula, the dose of heparin should be adjusted. Bandages should be applied to the puncture sites after the bleeding has stopped.

CATHETER CARE

Infections are likely to occur with catheters. Because of this, aseptic technique must be used when starting and ending a dialysis treatment. On starting or ending a dialysis treatment, the caps and ports of the catheter must be sterilized using a disinfectant-soaked cloth. The manufacturer provides instructions on the care of the catheter and the type of disinfectant that should be used to keep it clean. The caregiver must follow the manufacturer's instructions to ensure that the catheter remains intact and undamaged. The site where the catheter leaves the body must be cleaned with a disinfectant recommended by the dialysis facility after each dialysis treatment. The wound should be covered with a sterile dressing. If the exit site is red or if discharge is evident, it is indicative of an infection. After a dialysis treatment, heparin is introduced into the catheter port. The heparin is removed before the next treatment.

VASCULAR ACCESS CARE BETWEEN TREATMENTS

Enough heparin must be maintained inside the lumen of the catheter to prevent blood clots from forming, but heparin must be prevented from entering the patient's blood circulation. After a dialysis treatment, the catheter lumen must be cleared of blood cells by introducing 10 mL of normal saline. After the saline has been introduced into the lumen, 5000 units/mL of heparin must be rapidly instilled into the lumen. Rapid instillation is necessary so that the saline and heparin don't mix. The heparin will displace the saline in the catheter. After the heparin has replaced the saline in the catheter, the catheter lumen is clamped. Although the use of 5000 units/mL of heparin is standard, some dialysis facilities prefer to use 1000 units/mL.

AV FISTULA-RELATED COMPLICATIONS

PROBLEMS WITH THE AV FISTULA

Each hemodialysis treatment requires the insertion of a needle. Chronic hemodialysis requires repeated venipunctures. Over time, the tissue over the site of needle insertion becomes scarred. This scarring makes it more difficult to penetrate the tissue with the needle and the process becomes more painful for the patient. If the needle becomes displaced and infiltrates the vessel, a hematoma may develop in the fistula. The hematoma results when the vessel bleeds into the surrounding tissue. The swelling associated with an infiltration may make it impossible to use the fistula for access until the swelling subsides. After each hemodialysis treatment is finished the needles are withdrawn. Pressure must be applied over the site of the needle puncture for 10-20 minutes to control bleeding.

PROBLEMS WITH ACCESSING THE AV FISTULA

The vein used in an AV fistula must enlarge sufficiently so that the large-gauge needles used in dialysis can be inserted into the vein easily. This process of enlargement may take weeks or months. The process of vein enlargement takes longer in women than it does in men. The distribution of veins and arteries and the size of these vessels vary among individuals. It may be difficult to find appropriate vessels, making it necessary to reuse a few sites repeatedly. It is sometimes difficult to obtain the required blood flow. This may be due to the size of the veins, or to the diversion of blood flow by the branches. With side-to-side arteriovenous fistulas, the dilation can occur over the back of the hand instead of in the arm veins. This situation may require surgical correction.

SPASMS OF AN AV FISTULA

Blood vessels may spasm during a dialysis treatment. When a spasm occurs, it is often at the beginning of the hemodialysis treatment. Spasms of the vessels are common and usually occur with increased rates of blood flow when the fistula has not matured sufficiently. Spasms may occur when suction is created, causing the lumen of the needle to pull against the walls of the blood vessel. Suction between the needle and wall of the vessel can be painful for the patient. This occurrence can cause the needle to feel as if it were fluttering. The situation may be prevented by the use of back-eye needles. Spasms of the vessels interfere with blood flow and cause a decrease in the arterial blood flow.

THROMBOSES

Thrombosis is the complication that occurs most frequently in individuals with AV fistulas. Thrombosis in an individual with an AV fistula can be caused by infection, hypotension, and stenosis of the AV fistula. A stenosis is a narrowing of the fistula. There is a positive relationship between the percentage of stenosis and the occurrence of thrombosis. Thrombosis can also occur from an impeded blood flow. Tight bandages, a fistula needle device, lying on the fistula arm, and hematoma can interfere with blood flow and cause thrombosis. If 2 fistula-needle-holding devices are used simultaneously, this can encourage the development of thrombosis by cutting off circulation. After the placement of a fistula-needle-holding device or clamp on the access, the operator should determine that appropriate sounds can be heard on auscultation.

INFECTIONS AND ANEURYSMS

Infections and aneurysms are complications that can also occur with AV fistulas.

- **Infections** at the access site may result from inadequate care of the access site or from contamination during cannulation. Infection originally localized to the fistula site may result in thrombosis or sepsis. Infection may be demonstrated by redness, swelling, pain at the access site, and fever. If an infection is suspected, it is confirmed by blood culture or by culturing the drainage from the access site.
- An **aneurysm** is a bulging weakness in the wall of a blood vessel. Aneurysms can occur with an arteriovenous fistula for two main reasons: repeated cannulations from the same fistula, or infection.

COLLATERAL CIRCULATION

The redirection of the arterial blood through the vein eventually results in the thickening of the walls of the vein and the dilation of the vein. The process is called **maturation**. Maturation occurs due to the increased pressure in the vein caused by the arterial blood and the increased volume in blood flowing through the vein. The vein involved in the arteriovenous fistula sometimes develops new branches. These branches eventually enlarge and develop thickened walls, becoming mature. When mature, these branches can be cannulated, supplying additional access for dialysis. This formation of new branches of the vein that can be used in dialysis is called collateral circulation. Sometimes the collateral circulation prevents the maturation of the primary vein. If this occurs, the new branches must be ligated. It may take up to 4 months for an arteriovenous fistula to mature enough to allow cannulation.

RADIAL ARTERY STEAL SYNDROME

Radial artery steal syndrome involves ischemic changes in the fingers. Signs and symptoms of the syndrome include pain in the fingers and palm, coldness, and impaired function. In severe cases gangrene and necrosis are seen. The syndrome is caused by poor circulation to the hand and fingers. It occurs as a result of the creation of the fistula, which diverts the arterial blood into the vein. The radial artery and the ulnar artery are usually connected. Because of the fistula, this connection is disrupted. An abnormal pressure gradient causes the blood from the ulnar artery to flow toward the fistula instead of toward the fingers. The symptoms of radial artery steal syndrome worsen during a dialysis treatment. The situation can be corrected if treated promptly. To correct the syndrome, the radial artery is tied off distal to the fistula.

RECIRCULATION AND BLACK BLOOD SYNDROME

Recirculation results when the fistula has a low blood flow rate. This is an undesirable state and may be caused by stenosis. The stenosis is usually found in the venous end, but may occur in the arterial end. Recirculation and increase in venous pressure occur together. If the recirculation is severe enough, it may cause black blood syndrome.

Black blood syndrome is a term used to describe acidosis of the blood. This occurs in severe cases of recirculation. When the blood is acidotic, the cells are not able to carry sufficient oxygen. Acidotic blood has a low pH. The condition is called black blood syndrome because the blood takes on a dark appearance.

IMPROVING POOR BLOOD FLOW IN CATHETERS

If the blood flow with a subclavian or jugular catheter is not sufficient, it may be increased by lowering the patient's head or turning the head to the side opposite the catheter. External pressure may also be applied to the catheter's exit site. In the case of a catheter with wings, blood flow can be increased by rotating the shaft of the catheter 180 degrees. If nothing else works, blood flow may be sped up by reversing the catheter lines. This should be used only as a last resort.

Clotting occurs frequently with catheters. Clotting can be reduced if heparin is introduced into the catheter after dialysis according to the manufacturer's instructions. If the catheter is clotted, fibrinolytic agents may be used to dissolve the clot. Saline should not be introduced into the catheter to dislodge the clot. This may cause the clot to enter the bloodstream.

HEMOPERFUSION

Hemoperfusion is an extracorporeal treatment. Hemoperfusion is a process by which the blood is passed over an adsorbent material to remove toxic substances or waste substances. The adsorbent material may be packaged in the form of a cartridge or column. The adsorbent material used is often activated charcoal. The charcoal is covered by a polymer film, which serves to reduce the risk of embolism from the carbon particles. Hemoperfusion is a technique often used to treat drug overdose and exposure to toxic substances. The substances that hemoperfusion can remove from the blood include most sedatives, digoxin, and some pesticides and herbicides. The activated charcoal is able to bind most solutes in the range of 100-20,000 Da. Some cases of poisoning are best treated by hemoperfusion, but some substances are better removed by hemodialysis.

ADVERSE EFFECTS AND LIMITATIONS

Hemoperfusion may cause a transient reduction in platelets. This situation usually resolves within 24 hours. The white blood cell count may also decrease. Patients receiving hemoperfusion frequently become hypotensive, but the patient is already at risk for this because of his or her condition. Hemolysis and damage to the red blood cells is a rare occurrence.

There is a limit to the amount that the sorbent can absorb. Adsorption can be difficult to predict and its kinetics are not well understood. Clearance may decrease rapidly or gradually and this does not necessarily depend on the sorbent capacity of the material remaining. The transfer of material from the blood to the sorbent depends on the rate of fluid transfer and the rate of intraparticle transfer. These, in turn, are related to microcapillary size and solute diffusion.

HEMOFILTRATION

Hemofiltration is also called diafiltration. It is an extracorporeal mode of treatment and is a process by which waste products are removed from the blood. In hemofiltration, blood is passed by convective transfer across an extracorporeal filter. Hypotension occurs less often in hemofiltration than in hemodialysis. Hemofiltration rarely results in intracellular osmolar shift or disequilibrium. Hemofiltration leads to better blood pressure control between treatments than hemodialysis. Solutes of large molecular size can be removed. There are drawbacks to hemofiltration. The administration of replacement fluid must be monitored to prevent overhydration or underhydration. Blood leak is a very real danger and may occur with the use of negative pressure applied to the filtrate bag. Negative pressure is used to increase ultrafiltration. Hemofiltration may adversely affect blood levels of beneficial medications. Sterile replacement fluids are necessary and costly.

COLLECTING LABORATORY SAMPLES PRIOR TO TREATMENT

BLOOD SAMPLE TECHNIQUES

Collecting a blood sample involves withdrawing blood from a fistula needle or bloodline using a needle and syringe. If using the fistula needle, draw the sample before giving heparin or flushing. Remove the needle from an empty syringe. Draw the sample. Reattach the needle and push it through the rubber stopper on the evacuated blood tube. The hemodialysis technician can also use a Luer-Lok adapter to draw the blood directly into multiple blood tubes. When the blood stops flowing, the tube is full. Never try to force more blood into the tube. Adding too much blood makes the ratio of anticoagulant to blood incorrect. The blood may clot, the tube may crack, or the stopper may pop off, all of which make the sample unusable in the lab.

Use the same technique to draw blood from the injection port on the bloodline. Always cleanse the port per the unit's protocol before piercing it, to prevent contamination. This time, aspirate the blood with the needle attached.

POINTERS FOR DRAWING BLOOD WORK

Standard or universal precautions refer to the healthcare worker's responsibility to control the spread of disease by assuming that every patient's samples are infectious, and following the US Occupational Safety and Health Administration (OSHA) standards for proper hand washing, wearing gloves, bagging specimens in biohazard bags, and disposing of needles and lancets in an approved sharps safe. Always use standard precautions and aseptic technique when obtaining blood specimens. Draw the samples from the arterial needle or the bloodline injection port after proper disinfection. Draw blood work before giving any anticoagulant or saline. Draw lab tubes that contain anticoagulants last. Dispose of needles into approved sharps containers immediately after use. Invert the tubes gently several times to mix the blood with tube additives. Never shake the blood, as hemolysis results. Stand the tubes upright in a rack. Ensure samples are properly labeled with the patient's name, unique identifier, birthdate, and initials and the time. Keep specimens at the correct temperature (on ice, hot water bath, refrigerator, or room temperature) per protocol.

CENTRIFUGE

A **centrifuge** is the spinning device that causes cells or formed elements to settle in a pellet at the bottom of a tube and liquid supernatant to float on top. Blood separates as into the following:

- **Plasma**: Straw-colored liquid portion of unclotted blood.
- **Serum**: Clear liquid separated from clotted blood.

Examples of tests requiring centrifugation include the following:

- Microscopic urinalysis
- Hematocrit
- Antibody titers
- Plasmacrit test (PCT) for syphilis
- Virus isolation and identification
- Concentrated mycobacterial specimen for primary culture

The procedure for using a centrifuge is as follows:

1. Keep tubes upright 10—20 minutes before centrifugation.
2. Use standard precautions (gloves and goggles).
3. Open stoppers. If clot sticks, rim with heparin stick.
4. Parafilm tube tops to prevent inhaling aerosols.
5. Balance an equal number of tubes with equal volumes. An unbalanced centrifuge set for the wrong number of rotations traps plasma and produces erroneous results.
6. Set centrifuge for correct time and rotations (g).

Remember to never open a spinning centrifuge. Use the brake if glass shatters. Remove broken glass with forceps. Autoclave centrifuge cups. Vacuum out machine and clean with 95% ethanol.

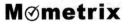

TIMING OF BLOOD SPECIMEN COLLECTION

Knowing when to take a blood sample is as important as the process of correctly obtaining it. Different hormones peak and trough at specific times during the day. The attending physician and microbiologist schedule the patient's next antibiotic dose with the nurse according to pre and post blood levels the hemodialysis technician obtains at specified times. Draw pre-dialysis blood samples after the patient has been cannulated, but before any heparin or flushes have been given. Check clotting time pre-dialysis. When blood is needed to measure the concentration of a substance in the patient's bloodstream, such as a drug level, then draw the sample from the arterial needle or the arterial bloodline. Draw post-dialysis specimens immediately after dialysis. Dialyzer clotting time is drawn post dialyzer. Kt/V tests to calculate uremic samples require a special technique.

COMMON LABORATORY TESTS IN PATIENT DIAGNOSIS AND MANAGEMENT

Numerous laboratory tests are used to monitor dialysis patients. Acceptable values for patients on dialysis have been established. These values may lie outside the values established in the general population. Values inappropriate to a dialysis patient may necessitate physician intervention, including a change in dialysis prescription. The following levels are monitored on an ongoing basis:

Sodium	Reticulocytes	Albumin
Potassium	Platelets	Total Protein
Chloride	Hematocrit	Cholesterol
Carbon Dioxide	Iron-Binding Capacity	Alanine Transaminase
Calcium	Phosphorus	Aspartate Transaminase
Creatinine	Magnesium	Blood Urea Nitrogen
Hemoglobin	Parathyroid Hormone	Ferritin
Iron	White Blood Cells	Aluminum
Glucose		

DRAWING THE PRE-DIALYSIS BLOOD SAMPLE FOR KT/V

Kt/V is a measurement of the dialyzer's clearance of urea. A high Kt/V is associated with better patient outcomes and decreased mortality and morbidity. The samples for Kt/V calculations must be drawn in a precise, consistent manner. All staff must use exactly the same technique each time they draw a Kt/V sample to ensure reliable results that can be compared over time. Draw the sample from a graft or fistula directly from the fistula needle, before any heparin or saline is given. If the patient uses a catheter for dialysis, first aspirate the heparin prime from the catheter, and then attach a new syringe and withdraw 10 cc of blood from the catheter. This ensures that no heparin mixes with the sample. Connect a new syringe to the arterial limb of the catheter to draw the sample. Kt/V is used with URR to determine adequacy.

SERUM CREATININE AND CREATININE CLEARANCE

Serum creatinine is a renal function test that is a very specific indicator of kidney function because it is not affected by changes in the fluid status of the patient, like the BUN level is. Creatinine is relative to muscle mass: A tall, muscular man will have a higher creatinine level than a small, thin woman. Changes in creatinine indicate a change in muscle mass and nutritional status. The normal level of serum creatinine for a pre-dialysis patient is anywhere from 10-18 mg/dL, but serum creatinine alone does not dictate the need for dialysis.

The 24-hour creatinine clearance test determines if kidneys are damaged by measuring their output of creatinine against the blood level. If the kidneys do not filter properly, creatinine output in the urine decreases, and blood level increases.

- Normal male: 95-104 mL/min
- Normal female: 95-125 mL/min
- Normal BUN to Creatinine ratio: between 10:1 and 20:1

BLOOD UREA NITROGEN (BUN)

Blood Urea Nitrogen (BUN) is a nitrogenous waste by-product of amino acid metabolism. Urea is the end product. BUN is normally excreted by the kidneys. The normal level is 7-18 mg/dL. Ammonia, BUN, urea, and creatinine are the renal function studies. High creatinine (over 1.5 mg/dL) and BUN (over 20 mg/dL) means the patient has kidney diseases like glomerulonephritis, pyelonephritis, stones, tubular necrosis, or tumors. Patients with ESRD have BUN levels between 60-100 mg/dL. BUN is usually monitored on a monthly basis. Causes of BUN elevation include a high protein diet, GI bleeding, fever, trauma, infection, or inadequate dialysis. Signs and symptoms of elevated BUN levels include sleeplessness, malaise, nausea, dry and itchy skin, changes in temperament, and distortions in taste and smell. BUN levels drop when using the antibiotics tobramycin or gentamycin, overhydration, liver failure, pregnancy, and shock.

ALBUMIN

Albumin is the most abundant protein found in the plasma. It is produced in the liver. Albumin helps to maintain fluid levels in the blood vessels. Albumin transports molecules in the blood (e.g., hormones, bilirubin, calcium, drugs). Serum albumin level is a useful measure of protein stores and is useful in the measurement of nutritional status. Low albumin levels will cause fluid to seep from the blood vessels into the surrounding tissue. Symptoms of low albumin (hypoalbuminemia) include weight loss, fatigue, low blood pressure, and muscle wasting. Hyperalbuminemia indicates severe dehydration. Albumin levels in the patient with end-stage renal disease can be used to predict morbidity and mortality. Albumin values in the blood range from 3.5-5.4 g/dL in the general population. Among individuals with end-stage renal disease, a value of greater than 4 g/dL is desirable.

C-REACTIVE PROTEIN (CRP) AND ALBUMIN LEVELS

CRP is a plasma protein produced by the liver in response to infection, acute inflammation, and tissue damage. In dialysis patients, **higher serum CRP is associated with low serum albumin.** These 2 factors in combination indicate that the patient is at high risk for heart disease and vasculitis (inflammation of the blood vessels). In a healthy individual, the level of serum CRP is usually less than 5 mg/L. Infection or trauma causes this level to increase significantly. A bacterial or viral infection can cause serum CRP to increase 100 times the normal level or more. CRP can be used to determine the presence of infection at an early stage. Levels of CRP are at their highest 2-3 days after the start of an infection. These levels start to decrease 1-2 weeks after the infection clears the system.

REASONS FOR LOW ALBUMIN

Diet affects the level of albumin in the bloodstream. Patients on dialysis may have low albumin levels due to a loss of appetite causing poor nutritional status. Uremia causes poor appetite. **Dialysis patients may not get adequate levels of protein for the following reasons**:

- Lack of knowledge regarding what constitutes adequate protein intake
- Difficulties with cooking or grocery shopping

- Nausea
- Loss of appetite for foods containing protein

Albumin may be excreted and lost in the urine. Albumin may also be lost during peritoneal dialysis when the protein is carried across the peritoneal membrane. Low albumin in the dialysis patient is associated with higher rates of hospitalization. It is also a reliable predictor of mortality. The risk of morbidity and death increases when serum levels of albumin drop below 3.5 g/dL.

COMPLETE BLOOD COUNT (CBC)

A complete blood count (CBC) is measured in the hematology laboratory. CBC checks for anemia, infection, and immune function. The doctor orders a CBC for the patient with kidney disease at least monthly and on an as-needed basis (PRN). Draw a lavender stoppered tube containing EDTA for the lab. CBC includes:

- White blood cell count (WBC) to detect infection or decreased immune functioning.
- Red blood cell count (RBC) for anemia.
- Hemoglobin (Hgb or Hb) for anemia.
- Hematocrit (Hct) for anemia.
- Differential (optional) to measure different types of WBC associated with particular problems, such as eosinophils for allergies.
- Erythrocyte sedimentation rate (ESR, optional) for severe bleeding, infection that would hamper the patient's response to Epogen, and parasite infestation

ANEMIA LABORATORY INDICATORS

Anemia is defined as a deficiency in red blood cells.

- **Physiology**: Patients with ESRD cannot produce erythropoietin hormone in their kidneys to stimulate new red blood cell (RBC) production in bone marrow. The normal RBC lifespan is 120 days, but the lifespan of RBCs in patients with renal disease is dramatically shortened because of phospholipids asymmetry.
- **Signs and Symptoms**: Decreased endurance, SOB, hypothermia, chest and abdominal pain, tachycardia, and depression.
- Anemia tests in complete blood count (CBC) include:
  - **Hematocrit (Hct)**: Percentage by volume of packed red blood cells in whole blood. Indirectly measures RBC mass. If RBCs are normal size, then Hct confirms RBC count. Patients with anemia and small RBCs do not have parallel Hct and RBC counts. This is reported as packed cell volume (PCV).
    - ❖ Normal values: Males 42-52%; females 36-48%
    - ❖ Levels commonly seen in ESRD: 30-36%
  - **Hemoglobin (Hb)**: Measures oxygen carrying capacity of RBCs.
    - ❖ Normal values: 12-16 g/dL (7.4-9.9 mmol/L)
    - ❖ Levels seen in ESRD: 11-12 g/dL
- **Treatment**: Epogen and blood transfusions.
- **KDOQI guidelines**: Individuals with stage 5 CKD should be monitored every 3 months for anemia. Individuals with stage 4 CKD should be monitored twice annually. Individuals with stage 3 CKD should be monitored annually. If a patient with CKD has been diagnosed with anemia, they should be routinely monitored at least every 3 months (or monthly in those with stage 5 CKD).

TRANSFERRIN TESTING

Transferrin is a protein that carries iron. It is produced in the liver. A transferrin protein carrying iron binds to a transferrin receptor on a cell surface and is transported in the form of a vesicle into the cell. Once inside the cell, the iron is released. Transferrin saturation (TSAT) is a measure of the amount of iron that can be used immediately in red blood cell production. It is calculated by dividing the iron concentration by the TIBC (total iron-binding capacity). The Kidney Disease Outcomes Quality Initiative guidelines recommend that patients with end-stage renal disease maintain a TSAT level above 30%. Serum transferrin levels can be used to check for both iron deficiency and disorders involving iron overload.

> **Review Video: Transferrin**
> Visit mometrix.com/academy and enter code: 267479

FERRITIN TESTING

Serum ferritin level is used to assess iron availability in individuals with end-stage renal disease. Ferritin is a protein in the body. Most of the ferritin in the body is stored in the liver, spleen, muscles of the skeleton, and bone marrow. Ferritin is found in small amounts in the blood. Ferritin stores iron and the amount of ferritin present in the blood is a measure of the amount of iron in the blood. Low ferritin levels indicate low iron levels. It is recommended in the Kidney Disease Outcomes Quality Initiative guidelines (2012) that serum ferritin level be maintained at a level greater than 100 ng/mL and less than 800 ng/mL in patients with end-stage renal disease. Serum ferritin level is considered the best measure for iron deficiency. It is also used to test for iron overload. Organ damage can raise ferritin levels.

CHR TESTING

CHr measures **reticulocyte hemoglobin content**. It is a test used to determine if an iron deficiency is present. It is also used to monitor the effects of iron therapy delivered intravenously. Reticulocytes are newly formed red blood cells. After being released into the bloodstream, reticulocytes circulate for 1-2 days. CHr is a measure of the amount of iron available to the most recently produced blood cells. For this reason, it provides a good measure of fast changes in iron availability. This test may be more informative than serum iron, ferritin, or transferrin saturation. CHr specifically indicates the iron content of the reticulocytes. This test can be used to determine the dose that should be used in intravenous iron therapy.

HEPATITIS TESTS

Patients in ESRD who are anemic have frequent blood transfusions and are at greater risk for developing hepatitis. The following tests are collected to monitor hepatitis in the patient with ESRD:

- **Hepatitis core antibody (HbC Ab)** is monitored twice per year. A positive test result means that the patient was exposed to Hepatitis B in the past.
- **Hepatitis B surface antibody (HbSAb)** is measured twice per year. If the patient was immunized against Hepatitis B, then he/she will have a positive result and is immune to Hepatitis B.
- **Hepatitis B surface antigen (HBsAg)** is measured monthly unless the result is positive. HBsAg is the earliest indicator that the patient has acquired an acute Hepatitis B infection.
- **Hepatitis C Antibody (anti-HCV)** is measured once per year. The expected result is negative. A positive result means the patient has acquired Hepatitis C and may transmit the virus.

Use blood precautions and isolation technique for patients with positive test results: Gown, glove, goggles, and 0.6% sodium hypochlorite (Javex) for disinfecting surfaces.

ALUMINUM LEVELS

Aluminum is widespread in the environment, and is found in tea, water, cookware, beverage and food containers, antacids, and antiperspirants. The kidneys are the main organs of elimination for aluminum. Aluminum deposits in the brain, tissues, and bone of dialysis patients. Aluminum toxicity was once more prevalent than it is today because antacids containing aluminum were used as binders to control phosphorus levels. High levels of aluminum cause bone disease and neurological problems, such as dementia, speech difficulties, and behavioral disorders. There is circumstantial evidence that aluminum deposits in the brain cause Alzheimer's disease. High aluminum levels can prevent Epogen from stimulating erythropoiesis (red blood cell production). Normal levels for aluminum in the serum are 0-10 mcg/L.

GLUCOSE

Glucose is blood sugar. Patients with low renal threshold or diabetes spill glucose in their urine. Fasting glucose level for the general population is 65-100 mg/dL. If the patient with kidney disease is not diabetic, measure serum glucose on a monthly basis. If the patient has well-controlled diabetes, measure the serum glucose level at the beginning of every dialysis treatment. If the patient has uncontrolled diabetes, then more frequent checks may be necessary, per doctor's order. There is glucose in the dialysate, so the patient's response must be monitored carefully for complications. Monitor for flushed skin, sleepiness, and heavy snoring that may lead to coma. Patients with ESRD metabolize insulin differently than normal patients. If the patient's blood sugar test result is below 50 mg/dL, notify the nurse. A 50 mL bolus of 50% dextrose may be needed to prevent progression to hypoglycemic shock. Elevated glucose levels may require the nurse to administer regular insulin to prevent diabetic coma.

HEPARIN ADMINISTRATION

For **intermittent intravenous administration of heparin**, an activated clotting time test is first conducted. Clotting time is normally 60-90 seconds. A priming dose of heparin, usually 25-50 units per kg of the patient's body weight, is then administered intravenously at the start of the dialysis treatment. During the procedure, smaller doses of heparin are administered at intervals. The goal of intermittent intravenous heparin administration is to keep the activated clotting time at approximately 3 times the activated clotted time determined at baseline.

For **continuous infusion of heparin**, after the administration of a priming dose of heparin, a bolus of about 2000 units is administered, and then the drug is infused at a constant rate throughout the treatment at a rate of 500 units per hour. The rate of clotting is evaluated at regular intervals and the dosage of the drug is adjusted as necessary. The administration of the drug is stopped 30 minutes to one hour before the treatment is scheduled to finish.

DOSAGE

Dialysis uses heparin in a concentration of 1000 units/mL. The same degree of anticoagulation is produced by the same number of units of beef lung or porcine mucosal heparin. The international unit used in Europe is slightly different from the USP unit. The heparin dose prescribed to each patient is based on his or her dry weight. The dose of heparin being used may need to be adjusted if the patient gains or loses weight. A change in the length of the treatment prescribed and changes in the dialyzer membrane may also necessitate a change in the heparin dosage. Erythropoietin may necessitate an increase in the amount of heparin administered. The dosage of heparin used must be high enough to prevent the blood from clotting in the extracorporeal circuit, but low enough that bleeding is not a problem.

Low-Dose Heparinization

Low-dose heparinization is also referred to as tight heparinization. This type of heparinization requires constant monitoring of the patient's clotting time. Only enough heparin is administered to maintain an activated clotting time of 90-120 seconds. Low-dose heparinization is the safest and most practical way of administering heparin if the patient is at risk of bleeding. Patients at risk for bleeding include those who are menstruating and recent surgical patients. Patients who are having their central line removed after treatment are also at risk for bleeding. The baseline clotting dose is first determined, and this provides the basis for the priming dose and the maintenance dose. Some dialysis facilities use low-dose heparinization for first-time dialysis patients.

Regional Heparinization

Regional heparinization is a technique in which an anticoagulant is introduced at a constant rate into the arterial bloodline while at the same time an antidote to the drug is introduced into the venous line. The arterial bloodline is the inlet of the dialyzer. The venous bloodline is the outlet through which the blood returns to the patient. Trisodium citrate is used as the antidote to the heparin. This substance acts in the extracorporeal circuit to bind the ionized calcium. The process of clot formation is dependent upon the presence of calcium ions. The dialysis fluid must not contain any calcium. Reinfusing the patient with blood that has decreased ionized calcium can cause harm. Therefore, calcium chloride is infused into the venous bloodline to reverse the condition.

Hemodialysis Without the Use of Heparin

Patients at risk for bleeding, pericarditis, clotting deficits, or thrombocytopenia can benefit from **heparin-free dialysis**. There are a number of techniques that can be used in heparin-free dialysis.

- The dialyzer unit, arterial bloodline, and venous bloodline are primed with a saline and heparin mixture. The heparin concentration in this solution is 3000 units of heparin/L. This solution is then drained from the dialyzer and bloodlines and discarded. If the patient is very likely to bleed, heparin is not used in the priming solution.
- The blood flow rate is set to be as rapid as can be tolerated by the patient.
- The dialyzer is rinsed frequently with 100-200 mL of saline. This procedure involves blocking the arterial bloodline and rapidly infusing the saline solution.

Identifying a Patient Prior to Treatment

The hemodialysis technician must identify the patient before beginning the dialysis process to ensure the following are confirmed:

- The right patient
- The right time
- With the right chemicals

Take the time to perform these checks to prevent serious errors:

- Even if the hemodialysis technician knows the patient well, they must always ask the patient to state his/her name. Ask him/her to spell the name if it is unclear or similar to another patient's. If there are two patients with the same name, check their birthdates, flag their charts and chairs, and separate them in different rooms, if possible. If the patient cannot talk or does not understand the languages spoken fluently, ask a caregiver who knows the patient. Utilize a medical interpreter for patients that cannot speak English.
- Look at the patient's chart to be certain that the most recent orders for the right patient are being used.
- Verify the name on the dialyzer with the patient or caregiver.
- Double check medications to be administered during dialysis for names and orders before the nurse gives them.

CHARTING PATIENT TREATMENT

The patient's chart is a legal document of the events and procedures carried out during a dialysis treatment. It is a subpoenable court document that explains what care the patient did or did not receive. For paper charting, always write in dark blue or black ink in the chart, never in pencil. Do not make erasures; rather strike the entry through and initial these changes. Never write derogatory comments about the patient or other staff in the patient's chart. Charting is a method of communication between staff members about the patient, and it provides continuity of care from shift to shift. The chart is a diagnostic aid and the foundation upon which decisions are made concerning changes in medical therapy. The patient's chart also provides data for infection control, risk management and quality control purposes, and is subject to inspection by various regulating bodies, such as Medicare. Understand the unit's policies regarding charting practices.

PROPER CHARTING TECHNIQUES

All entries in a patient's chart must follow the **FACT system** and be:

- **F**actual—Clearly describe the patient's complaints, such as a report of pain that includes its specific location, quality (sharp and stabbing or dull ache), duration, and medications taken to relieve it.
- **A**ccurate—Entries are legible and in ink when on paper. Never use correction fluid or an eraser. Draw a single line through the mistake. Write 'error' beside it and one's name and title or initials, according to unit policy.
- **C**omplete—Never leave lines completely or partially blank. Place a single line through it to prevent someone else from adding to the line.
- **T**imely—Include the time on all entries.

HIPAA requires the hemodialysis technician to maintain confidentially of all patient records. Release information on a need-to-know basis only. Never leave a paper chart or computer screen open to prying eyes. Report to the charge nurse, IT, and security if approached by the press, an insurance company, or suspicious persons. Secure one's password. Log off after each session.

> **Review Video: HIPAA**
> Visit mometrix.com/academy and enter code: 412009

Evaluate, Intervene, and Manage Treatment: During Treatment

PATIENT MONITORING DURING DIALYSIS

Many members of the dialysis team are involved in the monitoring of a patient receiving a dialysis treatment, including the hemodialysis technician, nurses, and patient care technicians. The role and responsibilities of the patient care technician is directed by and varies by each state. A patient is monitored on a continual basis by the appropriate dialysis personnel. Arterial pressure, venous pressure, rate of blood flow, transmembrane pressure, volume of ultrafiltrate removed, temperature of dialysis fluid, rate of flow of dialysis fluid, and conductivity of dialysis fluid are monitored on a continuous basis by machines. Dialysis personnel also keep track of the length and progression of the dialysis treatment. The general condition of the patient must be noted to include the patient's physiologic state, physiologic response to treatment, and vital signs. The patient may experience nausea, respiratory difficulties, agitation, itching, muscle jerks, irrational behavior, or pain. Each patient has a unique response to dialysis, and any changes in response should be considered significant. Any clinical conditions observed must be entered on the patient's chart and reported to the physician.

GLUCOSE MONITORING

It has been estimated that 20-40% of patients starting dialysis treatments are diabetic. When dealing with a diabetic patient, the patient's serum glucose should be measured at the start of each treatment. Glucose level may be checked with a commercial reagent strip, such as Chemstick or Accu-Chek. If the patient is an unstable diabetic, then blood glucose level must be checked more frequently. If the patient's serum glucose level is less than 50 mg/dL, then it may be necessary to administer 50 mL of 50% dextrose to prevent the onset of hypoglycemic shock. If the patient's glucose level is too high, it may be necessary to administer insulin to prevent diabetic coma.

IDENTIFYING CHANGES IN THE PATIENT'S PHYSICAL STATUS

Changes in the patient's general physical state may indicate the patient is at risk for or experiencing any of the following complications, which must be reported:

Physical Change	Symptoms
Uremia	Rapid weight gain, generalized edema, confusion, shortness of breath, nausea, ammonia breath, and pruritis.
Anemia	Fatigue, general weakness, pallor, feeling cold, craving ice chips, and impaired mental status.
Left ventricular hypertrophy	Shortness of breath, weakness, and activity intolerance.
Pericarditis	Chest pain that worsens when reclining, fever, fatigues, hypotension, dysrhythmia, and cough.
Osteopenia/Osteoporosis	Increasing curvature of spine, aching joints, and fractures.
Amyloidosis	Joint pain, carpal tunnel syndrome, fractures, and bowel obstructions.
Neuropathy	Burning peripheral pain, numbness, general muscle weakness, poor ambulation, and erectile dysfunction.
Pruritis and/or hives	Severe generalized itching (may indicate hyperphosphatemia) and raised red welts (often indicates allergic response).

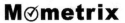

Physical Change	Symptoms
Insomnia/Sleep apnea	Frequent awakenings, difficulty falling or staying asleep, feeling of chronic fatigue and sleepiness.
Coagulopathy (clotting impairment)	Bleeding and/or bruising.
Stenosis of graft/fistula	Prolonged period of bleeding at the end of dialysis when needles removed.

IMPACT OF PHYSICAL CHANGES ON THE PATIENT'S COGNITIVE/MENTAL STATUS

Patients on dialysis have high rates (up to 70% in those ≥55 years) of cognitive impairment, especially because patients with chronic kidney disease on hemodialysis tend to have co-morbidities, such as hypertension, heart disease, stroke, and diabetes. Changes in a patient's cognitive/mental status may indicate the following, and must be reported:

Physical Change	Impact on Cognitive/Mental Status
Uremia	Patients often become confused and feel as though they are "in a fog."
Depression	Patients may become withdrawn, show little interest in activities, express negative feelings about disease and prognosis, and may appear confused at times.
Dialysis disequilibrium syndrome	In response to high levels of BUN, patients may exhibit a change in the level of consciousness as well as behavioral changes, or seizures, progressing to coma.
Hypotension	Patients may lose consciousness or experience frequent dizziness.
Seizures	Patients may exhibit a change in level of consciousness and may have a feeling of anxiety prior to the seizure.
Stroke	Patients may have sudden episodes of confusion and slurred speech (or inability to speak) and may have weakness on one side.
Delirium	Patients may exhibit rapid onset of fluctuating episodes of confusion and disorientation.

IDENTIFYING AND RESPONDING TO HEMODIALYSIS COMPLICATIONS

HYPOTENSION

Hypotension is the most common complication that occurs during hemodialysis. It occurs, in part, because ultrafiltration causes a decrease in blood volume. Hypotension can also result in dialysis patients due to poor vasoconstriction. Inadequate vasoconstriction can be caused by antihypertensive drugs and cardiac conditions. Ingesting food during a dialysis treatment can exacerbate hypotension by causing splanchnic vasodilation. This phenomenon is called postprandial hypotension, and it generally occurs approximately 2 hours after the patient has eaten. Because of the risk of postprandial hypotension and the accompanying potential for loss of consciousness, it is recommended that patients do not eat during a dialysis treatment. On occasion hypotension will occur in patients with small blood volumes. This occurs less frequently when smaller dialyzers are used.

60

TREATMENT

Although there are methods to prevent the development of hypotension during dialysis treatment, it still may occur. Hypotension may be caught early by monitoring the patient's blood pressure, by observing the patient, and by monitoring hemoglobin. The patient should be monitored so that if hypotension occurs, it can be treated in the early stages. **Early signs** of hypotension include lightheadedness, blurred vision, and upset stomach. If the patient complains of these symptoms, his or her blood pressure should be taken. Early hypotension can be treated by putting the patient in the Trendelenburg position, decreasing the rate of ultrafiltration, the administration of replacement fluids, or using a volume expander.

EDEMA AND HYPOTENSION

Some dialysis patients have severe edema due to heart failure or hypoproteinemia. Although the process of dialysis decreases the level of vascular fluid, fluid from the interstitial space is not removed. This is because the low level of protein in the blood does not exert the osmotic pressure necessary to remove the fluid. Some patients, who have no indications of cardiac failure or hypoproteinemia, become overhydrated during dialysis and this creates vascular instability. These individuals become hypotensive during dialysis and exhibit a rapid heart rate, nausea, and vomiting. The likely causes for this overhydration include changes in the osmolality of the blood, the actions of acetate (which may be used as a buffer), and the depletion of norepinephrine. The condition may be countered by infusions of hypertonic saline, the administration of mannitol, and a higher concentration of sodium in the dialysate. Sequential ultrafiltration may give better results.

ARRHYTHMIAS

Arrhythmias most often occur during dialysis due to an underlying cardiac issue. Arrhythmias occur most frequently in elderly dialysis patients. The patient's physician should inform dialysis personnel about any pre-existing heart disease. If the patient's heart rhythm alters during a dialysis treatment, an electrocardiogram should be conducted. The patient should be asked what medications he or she is taking. The patient's blood levels of potassium, calcium, and magnesium should be checked. Alterations in electrolytes may cause arrhythmias in patients with damage to the heart muscle.

If the patient with a heart condition develops chest pains during dialysis, angina should be presumed. The chest pain may be alleviated if the rate of blood flow is decreased or with the infusion of saline. **Nitroglycerin** taken before the dialysis treatment may prevent angina.

ALUMINUM TOXICITY

The kidneys filter and excrete aluminum taken into the body. Protein-bound aluminum is not easily removed by the kidneys as it does not diffuse easily through the glomeruli. If aluminum is taken into the body in large amounts, it is deposited in the bone and tissue. At one time, individuals on dialysis were exposed to high levels of aluminum. The water used in dialysis treatment contained aluminum, and aluminum-based phosphate binders were administered to the patients. This meant that patients were exposed to toxic levels of aluminum. The aluminum accumulated in the brain tissue, bone, and body tissues. High levels of aluminum in the body cause progressive neurological symptoms, such as slurred speech, memory loss, behavioral changes, and finally dementia. High levels of aluminum may also cause gastrointestinal irritation, loss of appetite, fatigue, anemia, and bone disease. Changes have been made to minimize aluminum exposure, but the risk still exists.

DIALYSIS AMYLOIDOSIS

Dialysis amyloidosis involves the production of an amyloid composed of beta-2-microglobulin. Normal kidneys excrete beta-2-microglobulin and prevent the buildup of this protein in the blood.

In patients with end-stage renal disease, the kidneys do not filter and excrete this protein. The treatment of patients with end-stage renal disease includes dialysis, but beta-2-microglobulin is poorly dialyzed, and builds up in the bloodstream. As the beta-2-microglobulin collects in the bloodstream, the molecules join together and form large molecules. These large molecules then deposit in the tissues of the body. The joints and periarticular structures are particularly affected. The condition causes great pain and limits motion, and can be progressive. Left untreated, it can be debilitating for the affected individual.

DEVELOPMENT AND TREATMENT

Individuals on dialysis for more than 3 years are likely to develop dialysis amyloidosis. Most patients who have been on dialysis for 10 years or longer will have dialysis amyloidosis. Dialysis amyloidosis is particularly common in adult patients. This complication of dialysis is less likely to develop in individuals dialyzed with high-flux synthetic membranes. More modern hemodialysis membranes and peritoneal dialysis remove beta-2-microglobulin more effectively than older hemodialysis membranes, but beta-2-microglobulin still accumulates in the blood. The beta-2-microgobulin is then deposited in bone, joints, and tendons. Hollow cysts may develop in the bone due to this deposition, leading to fractures. Amyloids deposited as a result of dialysis can also cause ligaments and tendons to tear.

MUSCLE CRAMPS

Cramps during dialysis can be **caused** by:

- Excessive fluid gain since the last treatment.
- Body weight gain, causing the removal of more fluid than needs to be attempted.
- Rapid shifts in blood components, especially the electrolytes sodium and potassium.
- Hypotension.

The hemodialysis technician makes the following **interventions** when the patient reports cramps:

- Counsel the patient about fluid gains between treatments.
- Carefully weigh the patient and assess for fluid gain pre-treatment.
- Ensure the correct dialysate is used, and sodium modeling parameters are as prescribed.
- Notify the patient's nurse of cramping.
- Make changes in the treatment plan per order, such as initiating a saline infusion; decreasing ultrafiltration rate, administering hypertonic saline, or changing the dry weight.

DIALYSIS DEMENTIA

Dialysis dementia, also called dialysis encephalopathy, is a syndrome experienced by individuals on chronic hemodialysis. The onset of the syndrome is not the same for all individuals. It may develop in individuals after several months, or several years, on dialysis. The signs and symptoms of the disease include confused and garbled speech, asymmetric muscle jerking, deterioration of mental processes, and convulsions. There are also characteristic brain wave patterns associated with the syndrome that can be seen on an EEG. Aluminum is suspected to be the cause of the syndrome in patients on dialysis. Calcium-containing phosphate binders are now being used instead of aluminum hydroxide and the syndrome has become much less common.

EXSANGUINATION

Risks for patient exsanguination (blood loss through their access site) relate to incorrect connection of the venous bloodline or separation of the line, dislodgement of the needle, ruptured dialyzer, rupture of fistula/graft, or failure to apply adequate pressure when needles removed.

Access site visibility is the most important factor. Because the blood is pumped through the system at the rate of 350 mL/min up to 500 mL/min, the patient can lose his or her total volume of blood within 10 minutes. While patient education is important, patients often fall asleep during treatment. Venous needle dislodgment is not always detected by alarms. HemaClips® are important safety additions, but should not replace observation. When removing hemodialysis needle after treatment, pressure must be applied to the access site for up to 20 minutes (varies according to patient) by using two fingers (not one) to apply pressure. The patient can be taught to apply pressure to the access sites but must be monitored while doing so.

AIR EMBOLISM

An air embolism involves the entry of air or microbubbles into the bloodstream. Air can get into the vascular system during dialysis and create an embolism when the bloodlines get disconnected from the dialyzer, or when the fluid in the blood or saline infusion bags runs out. The vacuum created by these occurrences causes the production of microbubbles. The air detector must be monitored by the dialysis personnel throughout the treatment. The symptoms of air embolism include chest pain, tightness in the chest, respiratory difficulties, and coughing. If air enters the cerebral venous system, the patient may exhibit neurological symptoms. Neurological symptoms caused by air embolism may include seizures, visual disturbances, and loss of consciousness.

TREATMENT

If the patient is showing signs and/or symptoms of an air embolism, immediate treatment is essential. The arterial and venous bloodlines must be clamped and the treatment stopped. The patient is then positioned on his or her left side into the Trendelenburg position. Placing the patient in this position helps prevent the embolism from moving to the brain. It slows the flow of air to the brain and traps any air present in the heart in the right atrium. This decreases the risk of foaming. Foam is produced largely in the right ventricle. The patient's airway must be kept open, and the movement of the patient should be kept to a minimum. The air will be reabsorbed, but it might take several hours. A chest-x-ray can determine the amount of air present in the heart.

HEMOLYSIS

Hemolysis is a term describing the breakdown of red blood cells. This process releases intracellular potassium. Chemical, thermal, and mechanical processes involved in dialysis can all cause hemolysis. The blood may be exposed to chemicals during dialysis. Hemolysis may result if the blood is exposed to sodium hypochlorite, formaldehyde, copper, or nitrates. Overheated dialysis fluid can cause hemolysis by heating the red blood cells. This can occur when the dialysis fluid is warmer than 42 °C. Hemolysis during dialysis can also have mechanical causes. These include kinked bloodlines, blocked blood pumps, the use of a small-gauge needle with high rates of blood flow, or a wrongly positioned needle. Hemolysis can be a chronic or acute occurrence. Incidents of hemolysis can range from a mild condition to a medical emergency.

SYMPTOMS

Hemolysis changes the appearance of the extracorporeal blood. It may appear transparent and cherry red in color, or opaque and very dark red in color. The patient may feel a burning sensation in the access arm. This burning occurs when the red blood cells rupture and release potassium in large amounts. There are numerous other symptoms associated with hemolysis. These include pain or cramping in the abdominal region, pain in the lower back or chest, nausea, vomiting, or respiratory distress. The potassium released from the breakdown of the red blood cells may cause an irregular, or abnormally rapid, heartbeat. The patient may become hypotensive or hypertensive. The hemoglobin levels drop quickly when the red bloods cells break down.

TREATMENT

Although the dialyzer monitors should detect problems that may cause hemolysis, these monitors can malfunction. The dialysis personnel should not depend entirely on the alarms, but should monitor the patient's physical condition. If the caregiver suspects hemolysis, he or she should clamp the bloodlines, stop the blood pump, and tend to the patient. This is essential to prevent a life-threatening situation from developing. The dialysis fluid should be tested for pH level and conductivity. The patient's blood should be tested for electrolyte levels, hemoglobin, and haptoglobin. The blood sample can be placed in a serum separator and centrifuged. In the case of hemolysis, the serum will be red. Hemolyzed blood should not be reinfused into patients as it can cause hyperkalemia.

DIALYZER REACTIONS

Dialyzer reaction is a term referring to a situation in which the patient exhibits allergy-like symptoms on first exposure to the dialysis membrane. Dialyzer reaction is sometimes called first-use syndrome. Dialyzer reactions are divided into two types called Type A and Type B. **Type A dialyzer reactions** are more severe than Type B dialyzer reactions. Type A reactions often involve symptoms of anaphylaxis. Symptoms of Type A reactions generally occur within 5 minutes after the start of treatment. Symptoms of Type A reaction include shortness of breath, chest pain, back pain, itching, hives, coughing, sneezing, watery eyes, a feeling of being warm, cramps in the abdominal region, and cardiac arrest. **Type B dialyzer reactions** are more common and less severe than Type A reactions. The symptoms start when the blood that has been exposed to the dialyzer is returned to the patient, generally within 15-30 minutes of the initiation of dialysis, although they may occur later. Type B symptoms include chest pain, back pain, and hypotension.

TYPE A DIALYZER REACTIONS

Type A dialyzer reactions are generally caused by a sterilant used in the factory. This sterilant is ethylene oxide. Type A reactions occur less often now because many dialyzer manufacturers are using other methods of sterilizing their product. If the manufacturer uses ethylene oxide to sterilize its dialyzers, priming of the dialyzer before first use may clear the sterilant from the unit.

The treatment for dialyzer reaction depends on the symptoms exhibited by the patient. As soon as the patient shows signs and symptoms of dialyzer reaction, the dialysis treatment should be stopped and the physician notified. The cause of the condition should be determined. If the patient is having breathing difficulties, oxygen should be administered. If the patient is showing signs of anaphylaxis, antihistamines or epinephrine may be administered.

FORMALDEHYDE REACTIONS

Formaldehyde is used as a sterilant. If the patient's blood is exposed to this sterilant, a formaldehyde reaction may occur. This situation occurs when the dialyzer is improperly rinsed and residual formaldehyde remains in the dialyzer. A patient with formaldehyde reaction may complain of dyspnea, a peppery taste in his or her mouth, a burning sensation from the venous needle, numbness in the face around the lips, and chest or back pain. Hemolysis of the red blood cells may occur with formaldehyde reaction. If symptoms of formaldehyde reaction are evident, the dialysis treatment should be stopped immediately. To ensure that the patient is not exposed to any more formaldehyde, 10 mL of blood should be taken out of each needle.

PYROGEN REACTIONS

A pyrogen is a fever-inducing substance. Although pyrogens are usually endotoxins, they can be exotoxins. In dialysis, pyrogens are usually endotoxins that form as byproducts of dead bacteria. Although bacteria themselves are too large to pass through the dialyzer membrane, endotoxins are smaller and can pass through the membrane. Symptoms of a pyrogen reaction include chills, fever, muscle pain, nausea, vomiting, and a drop in systolic blood pressure. When dialysis treatment is discontinued, the symptoms usually abate or disappear. The patient may need to be treated for hypotension and fever. It may be necessary to take blood cultures from the patient. As septicemia involves the same symptoms as pyrogen reaction, it must be ruled out as a cause of the patient's symptoms. Pyrogen reaction can be prevented by proper disinfection techniques and by not reusing dialyzers for longer than specified in the manufacturer's directions.

DISEQUILIBRIUM SYNDROME

Disequilibrium syndrome occurs shortly after a patient begins receiving dialysis treatment. The cause of the syndrome is unknown, but it produces neurological symptoms. It has been suggested that the syndrome results when a patient with an extreme case of uremia receives dialysis for the first time. As the urea is cleared from the patient's blood, the plasma becomes increasingly hypotonic. This causes the movement of water into the brain tissue from the plasma. The brain tissue is less hypotonic and contains a higher level of urea. The influx of water causes the brain tissue to swell. Symptoms include headache, nausea, vomiting, muscle twitching, muscle tremors, mental confusion, and seizures. Treatment includes the administration of a hypertonic solution, such as hypertonic saline, 50% dextrose, or mannitol. The symptoms of this syndrome can be minimized by using a less effective dialysis treatment until the levels of urea nitrogen in the blood are stabilized.

REVERSE FILTRATION

Reverse filtration occurs when the hydrostatic pressure in the fluid compartment is higher than the hydrostatic pressure in the blood compartment. This results in the movement of dialysis fluid from the fluid compartment into the blood compartment. The control mechanism of the ultrafiltration dialysis system uses reverse filtration to prevent the removal of an excessive amount of fluid. The pressure in the dialyzer is usually positive where the blood enters the dialyzer. This moves water and molecules from the blood compartment to the fluid compartment. If necessary, this gradient is reversed so that the pressure is negative toward the outlet. This moves fluid from the dialysis compartment into the blood compartment.

REVERSE DIALYSIS

Nonsterile water is used to make dialysis fluid. In addition, bicarbonate concentrate is added to the dialysis fluid and this substance promotes bacterial growth. Endotoxins from the dialysis fluid, as well as breakdown products, may enter the blood compartment from the fluid compartment in reverse dialysis. Pyrogen reactions may occur with reverse dialysis. Other adverse reactions may occur from reverse filtration. Measures can be taken to counter the adverse effects of reverse dialysis. A molecular filter positioned in the fluid delivery line can be used to remove suspended molecules while allowing dissolved solutes to pass through. Bacteria, pyrogen, and fragments of pyrogen cannot pass through the ultrafilter. The molecular filter is an ultrafiltration membrane.

CHILLS AND FEVER DURING DIALYSIS

Chills may or may not be accompanied by **fever**. If chills and fever are present before dialysis is initiated, it can indicate a viral or bacterial infection of the access, urinary tract, or respiratory infection. Chills that start after treatment is initiated and are accompanied by an increase in temperature could be caused by contamination of the dialyzer, bloodlines, dialysate, or the water treatment system. Chills without fever can indicate that the dialysate is too cold. Always check dialysate temperature prior to initiating treatment, and remember that 37 °C dialysate does not suit all patients. Patients with a cool body temperature benefit from cooler dialysate. 34 °C-35.5 °C improves hemodynamic stability. 35.5 °C improves heart contractility. Monitor the patient's vital signs closely, including temperature. Report chills and fever to the nurse. The physician will likely order a culture and sensitivity test. Assist with the collection of any lab specimens according to the unit's protocols.

SHOCK

Shock during dialysis usually results from a combination of hypotension and volume loss. Signs of shock during dialysis are a decrease in blood pressure, vomiting, incoherence, and unresponsiveness. The correct treatment sequence for shock is:

1. Check the patient for pulse and respirations.
2. If the patient has arrested (no palpable pulse), call Code Blue and initiate CPR. If the patient is still breathing, call the nurse for assistance.
3. Determine if the shock is due to excessive fluid removal or blood loss. Check the integrity of the access and dialyzer circuit. Is there blood on the floor or under the chair?
4. Place the patient in a left side-lying Trendelenburg position (head lower than feet to increase blood flow to the brain and reverse syncope). Cover the patient with a blanket to keep him/her warm.
5. Administer saline while monitoring blood pressure. Shock from excessive fluid removal should respond to the infusion of normal saline.

BLOOD LEAKS

The dialyzer compartment is a pressurized system. If the dialysis membrane ruptures during treatment, it allows blood to mix with dialysate. Dialysis machines have programmed detectors, which sense the presence of red blood cells in the outgoing dialysate effluent and sound an alarm. A large **blood leak** can cause the serum in the dialysate to turn pink. However, most leaks are invisible to the naked eye. Address all blood leak alarms, even if the fluid is yellow or clear, not pink. Check for the presence of blood in the dialysate effluent with a Hemastix reagent strip. If the dialysate is clear and no blood is detected with Hemastix, then resume dialysis after clearing the alarm. If the dipstick test is positive, stop treatment and do not return dialyzed blood to the patient. Patients with blood leaks develop abdominal, back and chest pain; SOB; nausea; vomiting; cyanosis; and diarrhea on average around 115-120 minutes after treatment begins.

CARPAL TUNNEL SYNDROME

Carpal tunnel syndrome is the compression of the median nerve in the carpal tunnel sheath of the wrist. Carpal tunnel syndrome develops in approximately half of individuals with dialysis amyloidosis. Carpal tunnel syndrome develops in these individuals as a result of the accumulation of proteins in the wrist. The carpal tunnel sheath becomes thickened by the deposits of amyloid and presses on the median nerve. The condition causes pain, numbness, and tingling in the thumb, index, and middle finger. The condition may be associated with muscle weakness in the hand. Carpal tunnel syndrome in individuals with dialysis amyloidosis can be treated by nonsteroidal anti-inflammatory medications and ultrasound treatments. The condition usually disappears after renal transplantation.

OXYGEN ADMINISTRATION DURING DIALYSIS

Oxygen may be administered to dialysis patients to increase the rate of oxygen in the blood and to decrease the risk of hypoxia, which leads to vasodilation and hypotension. Reducing the risk of hypotension is especially important because it is usually treated with a bolus of IV fluids and/or reduction of ultrafiltration rate, which can exacerbate fluid retention. Typical methods of administration include:

- **Nasal cannula**: Low-flow oxygen is usually administered at 2-3 L/min (maximum of 6 L/min) and oxygen saturation monitored. Oxygen per nasal cannula (prongs) delivers FiO_2 of 23-30% at 1-2 L/min and 30-40% at 3-5 L/min. Humidification should be used for prolonged flow rates >4 L/min. The cannula may cause nasal irritation.
- **Face mask**: Oxygen is usually administered at 6-8 L/min and delivers FiO_2 of 40-60%, but this may vary depending on how well-fitted the mask is to the patient.

ROLE OF HEMODIALYSIS TECHNICIAN IN PATIENT RESUSCITATION

The hemodialysis technician should be trained in CPR. They should immediately call for help from a nurse on duty if a patient goes into cardiac arrest and requires resuscitation and should initiate CPR until relieved by the nurse. The role of the hemodialysis technician may include:

- Positioning patient for CPR.
- Noting time of arrest and initiation of CPR.
- Verifying DNR status if applicable.
- Stopping the treatment and returning the blood to the patient if advised to do so.
- Flushing the lines with normal saline to provide IV access.
- Assisting with resuscitation efforts as directed by the nurse/physician.
- Pulling screens or curtains around patient station if available to ensure privacy.
- Obtaining the crash cart and AED or other necessary equipment.
- Monitor patient's peripheral pulse during compressions to assess for effectiveness.
- Recording treatments provided, including time.

MEASURING ACCESS RECIRCULATION

The slow stop-flow technique is used to measure access recirculation. The test is started after 30 minutes of treatment. The ultrafiltration device is then turned off. Arterial and venous blood samples are drawn from the inflow line and outflow line respectively. Blood flow rate is decreased to 50 mL/min. After the blood flow rate has been decreased, the blood pump is turned off. The arterial line is clamped above the sampling port. Systemic and/or peripheral blood samples are taken from the arterial port line. The arterial line is then unclamped and dialysis is resumed.

There are newer systems now in use to measure access recirculation. These include the HD03 hemodialysis monitoring system and the Crit-Line instrument.

HD03 HEMODIALYSIS MONITORING SYSTEM

The HD03 hemodialysis monitoring system (an upgrade of the HD01 system) is manufactured by Transonic Systems of Ithaca, New York. The system makes use of ultrasound technology and is based on saline dilution. This system monitors access recirculation with the use of flow dilution sensors. These sensors are attached to the arterial and venous bloodlines. To measure access recirculation, saline is introduced into the system by an injection through the venous drip chamber or through a port in the venous tubing. A computer and special program determine the percentage of access recirculation by measuring the level of flow through the arterial and venous bloodlines and alterations in the ultrasound signal speed. The Transonic Systems device can also measure cardiac output in patients.

CRIT-LINE

The Crit-Line monitoring instrument measures real-time hematocrit, blood volume levels/dilution, and oxygen saturation using an optical technique that is noninvasive. The Crit-line instrument involves a disposable blood chamber positioned between the arterial blood tubing and the dialyzer's arterial port. An optical sensor is connected to both the blood chamber and the Crit-Line device. Saline is then infused. The system **measures the percentage of access recirculation according to changes in hematocrit.**

RESPONDING TO PRESSURE MONITORS DURING DIALYSIS

Monitor the dialysis patient's pressures at least hourly during dialysis, or more frequently if mandated by unit policy. Talk to the patient to discreetly determine changes in consciousness. Frequent monitoring ensures that the patient is responding well and that machine parameters remain correctly set.

- **Arterial pressure measurement** records the pressure between the patient's needle site and a measurement site placed before the blood pump. Rising arterial pressure indicates clotting of the access or blood circuit, hypotension, a dislodged needle, or kink in the arterial line. Increases in negative pressure mean that blood flow to the machine is diminished. A prolonged high negative pressure causes hemolysis.
- **Venous pressure measurement** detects pressure post dialyzer, but before it returns to the patient's body. Increases in venous readings indicate clotting in the dialyzer or venous circuit, malpositioning of the needle, or a kink in the venous line. Decreases in venous pressure mean needle dislodgement, the transducer is wet, or the arterial chamber has clotted. Correct pressure alarms before resuming dialysis.

Evaluate, Intervene, and Manage Treatment: Post-Treatment

COLLECTING THE POST-DIALYSIS BUN SAMPLE

Draw the post-dialysis BUN sample at the end of treatment, before disconnecting the patient from the dialysis machine. Use either the slow flow or the stop pump technique. At the end of dialysis, turn the dialysate flow to the minimum setting or off. The arterial and venous pressure limits may need to be adjusted.

- **Slow flow technique**: Stop blood flow for 3 minutes, then draw blood from the arterial sampling port closest to the patient. Then discontinue treatment, per unit policy.
- **Stop pump technique**: Stop the blood pump after 15 seconds with the BFR at 100 mL/min. Clamp the arterial and venous lines and the arterial needle tubing. Obtain the sample from the arterial sampling port closest to the patient.

TERMINATING DIALYSIS TREATMENT WITH AV FISTULA OR GRAFT

After the dialysis treatment is completed, information recorded, and the lines all clamped, the needles are removed one at a time, generally starting with the distal needle first. The tape is removed from about the needle end, and a gauze pad is positioned over the needle so that pressure can be applied immediately as the needle is removed. After the hemodialysis needle is removed, the correct procedure is to apply pressure to the access site for up to 20 minutes (varies according to patient) by using two fingers (not one) to apply pressure. The patient can be taught to apply pressure to the access sites. The needles can be removed one at a time, allowing the first one to stop bleeding before doing the second, or the needles can be removed one after another, and the patient can apply pressure to one site and the technician to the other. Once all bleeding has stopped a bandage is applied over the insertion sites.

CARING FOR VASCULAR ACCESS AFTER DIALYSIS TREATMENT

The procedure for vascular access care post-treatment is as follows:

1. Remove the needles from the patient's access, taking care not to apply pressure before the needle is completely removed, as this may cause internal damage to the access.
2. Follow the RED rule: Rest, elevation, and direct pressure. Apply fingertip pressure over the needle site with sterile gauze. Exert enough pressure to stop the blood flow but not occlude the access. Encourage the patient to hold his/her own needle sites. Maintain pressure continuously for at least 10 minutes before checking for bleeding. Bleeding longer than 20 minutes can indicate access complications such as stenosis or the excessive administration of heparin. Always report bleeding that exceeds 20 minutes to the nurse in charge of the patient. Never place hemostat clamps on both needle sites at once, as clotting of the access could result.
3. After hemostasis is achieved, cover the needle sites with adhesive bandages.

Machine Technology

Maintain Dialysis Machine

THE DIALYZER

A dialyzer is an artificial kidney. The dialyzer is a filter designed to clear the blood of selected molecules, such as toxins and unwanted solutes. The dialyzer filters these toxins and unwanted solutes through a semipermeable membrane. A blood compartment is maintained on one side of the membrane and a compartment containing the dialysis fluid is maintained on the other side of the membrane. The delivery system of the dialyzer ensures that the dialysis fluid is of the proper temperature and of the correct chemical composition. The fluid and solutes are transferred through the processes of diffusion and convection. There are different types of dialyzers, but they all have a series of parallel flow paths to provide a large surface area between the blood and dialysis membrane and between the membrane and dialysis fluid.

HOLLOW-FIBER DIALYZERS

The most common dialyzer in use is the **hollow-fiber artificial kidney** (HFAK). HFAKs are manufactured in a wide range of sizes and with a wide range of membrane types. The semipermeable membrane of the HFAK comes in both cellulose and synthetic varieties. The membrane is comprised of very small, hollow fibers. These fibers range in diameter from 150-250 μm. The membranes also come in a variety of thicknesses. Some membranes may only be 7 μm thick, while others may be more than 50 μm thick. The hollow-fiber artificial kidney works by countercurrent flow. Countercurrent flow involves the flow of the blood and dialysate in opposite directions. This is considered to be a gentle form of dialysis.

ADVANTAGES AND DISADVANTAGES

The advantages of hollow-fiber dialyzers are as follows:

- Due to the flow geometry of the HFAK, the volume of blood contained in the dialyzer is low relative to the surface area of the dialyzer.
- There are a large number of passages resulting in low resistance to blood flow.
- HFAKs are not compliant.
- The rate of ultrafiltration can be regulated precisely.
- HFAKs can be reused.

The disadvantages of hollow-fiber dialyzers are as follows:

- The fiber bundle must be deuterated before starting the dialysis treatment or air lock may occur, preventing the entry of blood.
- The blood distribution may be uneven at the inflow header space, resulting in reduced perfusion in some of the center fibers.
- Ethylene oxide is used to sterilize HFAKs, and there may be residual toxic products after sterilization.

STERILIZATION

Hollow-fiber artificial kidneys are often sterilized with ethylene oxide. There may be toxic products left over after sterilization with this chemical. These residual toxic products may cause adverse reaction in some patients. There are other ways to sterilize hollow-fiber artificial kidneys. Gamma irradiation may be used by some manufacturers to sterilize these dialyzers. Steam sterilization is employed by other manufacturers. Both of these methods effectively sterilize HFAKs. HFAKs may be sterilized at the factory by electron beam (e-beam). This is a newer method of sterilizing HFAKs. The electron beam sterilization inactivates or destroys microorganisms by inducing a chemical reaction. The process does not use chemicals or radioactive materials, and is a good alternative to the use of ethylene oxide.

PARALLEL PLATE DIALYZERS

Parallel plate dialyzers are less commonly used and are arranged in layers. The layers are made up of supporting plates and sheets of membranes. The membranes are positioned in between the supporting plates. The plates are shaped to support the membrane and have ridges, grooves, or cross-hatches. These features also direct the flow of dialysate. The blood flows through the membrane sheets. The parallel plate dialyzer has drawbacks. The blood flow around the inlet port, outlet port, and corners may be uneven. This can lead to the formation of clots, resulting in the growth of bacteria and the formation of toxins. Therefore, plates are not typically reused. The dialyzer is also compliant, meaning that it can hold more blood as the TMP increases. There are also advantages to the parallel plate dialyzer. Because there is little clotting in the blood compartment, the requirement for heparin is generally low. Ultrafiltration can be regulated.

DIALYSIS MEMBRANES
SEMIPERMEABLE MEMBRANE

In dialysis treatment, the semipermeable membrane of the dialyzer permits some solutes to pass through for filtering, but does not allow all solutes through. The semipermeable membrane contains small pores through which some solutes can pass. Solutes that are too large to pass through the pores are retained. The ease with which solutes pass through the membrane is related to their size. Small molecules pass more easily through the membrane than larger solutes. When the patient's blood is directed through a compartment defined by the semipermeable membrane, particles small enough to pass through the pores enter the dialyzing fluid surrounding the compartment. For example, water, electrolytes, urea, creatinine, and glucose pass through the membrane by diffusion. Red and white blood cells, platelets, and the majority of plasma proteins cannot pass through the membrane.

CELLULOSE MEMBRANES

Cellulose is the organic structural material found in the cell wall of plants. It is a complex carbohydrate. The cellulose used in industry is generally obtained from wood pulp and cotton. Heat and chemical treatment turn the cellulose into a liquid slurry. After this substance coagulates, it is processed into sheets or hollow fibers. Membranes of different thickness and permeability are produced. Different processes produce membranes with different abilities to absorb water. The fibers making up the cellulose membranes swell when exposed to water. The pores of the membrane are complex tunnels that might be several times as long as the membrane is thick. Cuprophane is a cellulose material commonly used in the manufacturing of dialysis membranes. To form Cuprophane, the cellulose is treated with ammonia and copper oxide. Other cellulose materials used for dialysis membranes include saponified cellulose ester, cellulose acetate, and triacetate.

ADVANTAGES AND DISADVANTAGES

Cellulose membranes have been used in dialysis treatment for a significant period of time. The transport characteristics and other properties of these membranes are well understood. Cellulose membranes are fairly inexpensive relative to synthetic membranes. There is a disadvantage to the use of cellulose membranes. All types of cellulose membranes are incompatible with blood to a certain extent. Several studies have suggested that this factor can create significant problems. For example, cellulose acetate may be associated with a more rapid loss of residual kidney function than occurs with a synthetic type of membrane. In addition, it is thought that more compatible membranes lead to better recovery and survival rates. The improved recovery and survival rates associated with biocompatible membranes may be due to less complement activation, lower white cell activity, and less inflammation.

Cellulose acetate membranes have advantages. Membranes made of cellulose acetate are highly permeable to water. They are also inexpensive when compared to other membrane types. There are also disadvantages to cellulose acetate membranes. For example, they do not filter out low molecular weight solutes efficiently. This membrane type does not tolerate a wide range of pH levels. The membranes also break down if the temperature rises above 35 °C or 85 °F.

SYNTHETIC MEMBRANES

The synthetic material used in dialysis membrane is thermoplastic. These membranes are thin with a smooth surface. The supporting walls of the membrane are spongy. Because of their structure the walls of the membrane can trap contaminants. This can help protect the patient from the effects of these contaminants. The materials used in dialysis include polyacrylonitrile, polysulfone, polycarbonate, polyamide, and polymethyl-methacrylate. Synthetic membranes cause less of an inflammatory reaction than cellulose membranes. The ultrafiltration coefficients of synthetic dialysis membranes are 20-70 mL/hr per mmHg. Synthetic membranes are easily reused. There are disadvantages to synthetic membranes. They are expensive in comparison to cellulose membranes. It is necessary to use automated ultrafiltration because of the high water permeability of these membranes. The membranes may absorb proteins. There is a risk of back filtration due to the high permeability of the membranes.

The advantages of **polyamide membranes** include a tolerance to a wide range of pH levels. This type of membrane is more resistant to the actions of bacteria and withstands hydrolysis better than cellulose membranes. One of the disadvantages of polyamide membranes is that they are very susceptible to the actions of free chlorine and break down easily in the presence of this chemical.

THIN FILM COMPOSITE MEMBRANES

Membranes made of thin film composite have many advantages over other types of membranes, but they are expensive. These membranes are made of more than one type of material. The bottom layer of a thin film composite membrane is usually made of porous polysulfone. A layer made of a solute-rejecting material is attached to the bottom layer. This second layer is both thin and dense. It is often composed of polyfurane cyanurate or a polyamide. The thin film composite membrane is superior to the cellulose membrane in water flux and solute rejection. This type of membrane is less likely to compact than other types of membranes and is less susceptible to the adverse actions of bacteria.

CHLORINE-RESISTANT MEMBRANES

Chlorine-resistant membranes have a number of important advantages. Chlorine-resistant membranes are robust and long-lasting. They have a longer life than other types of membranes used in RO systems. These membranes can stand up to a wide range of pH levels. They can also tolerate diverse temperatures. Chlorine-resistant membranes also have a high water flux compared to other membranes. There is one main disadvantage to this type of membrane. The presence of divalent ions in the water adversely affects the rejection of monovalent ions. As a result, if a chlorine-resistant membrane is being used, it is necessary that the water fed into the RO system be softened or deionized first.

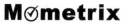

MEMBRANE BIOCOMPATIBILITY

The contact of blood with a foreign surface produces an inflammatory response. The strength of the inflammatory response is used to assess the biocompatibility of a dialysis membrane. An intense or a mild reaction may be elicited when blood comes into contact with the dialysis membrane. The dialysis membrane is considered to be bioincompatible when contact with it elicits an intense reaction and severe inflammation. The dialysis membrane is said to be compatible when the reaction and inflammation elicited are mild. The compatibility of the membrane has long and short-term repercussions. The intensity of the body's reaction to the membrane is determined after the start of hemodialysis. Complement activation is a measure of the severity of the response to the dialysis membrane. The markers used to assess complement activation are contained in the patient's blood. These markers are C3a, C5a, and C5b through C9.

COMPLEMENT ACTIVATION

The complement system is comprised of plasma proteins that react in sequence to defend the body when it is exposed to foreign substances. The dialysis membrane is perceived as a foreign substance. The first sign of complement activation in reaction to dialysis is leukopenia (an abrupt drop in white cell count). The leukopenia is transient in nature and the white count is at normal levels by the end of the treatment. Leukopenia can be dangerous for individuals with cardiac or pulmonary conditions. White cells are activated by the release of C5a. The activated white cells are sticky and can clump together in the capillary bed. The capillary bed in the lungs is often affected. This results in a reduction in pulmonary perfusion and a deficit in gas exchange. This can cause hypoxemia. Chest pain, back pain, abnormalities in coagulation, and anaphylaxis can also occur.

Because of its chemical composition, cellulose membranes and cellulose-based dialysis membranes are more likely to cause complement activation than synthetic dialysis membranes. The cellulosic surface is similar in composition to bacterial cell walls. The cell walls of bacteria and the surface of cellulose are both composed of chains of polysaccharides. The body reacts to cellulose in much the same way as it reacts to bacteria. The cellulose surface contains free hydroxyl groups and these are thought to be the main cause of the complement activation. The cellulosic membrane can be altered by buffering the free hydroxyl groups. This makes the cellulose membrane less likely to cause complement activation, but doesn't prevent it completely. An example of a modified cellulose membranes is cellulose acetate. Synthetic dialysis membranes do not have the reactive sites that create complement activation.

DISINFECTION PROCEDURES

STERILIZATION, DISINFECTION, AND CLEANING

Sterilization is meant for equipment that pierces the skin or contacts internal tissues. It kills all pathogens, including bacterial spores, and requires steam, dry heat, or ethylene oxide gas. If the item is too fragile for heat exposure, use an FDA-approved liquid sterilant at the recommended concentration for the required contact time.

Intermediate sterilization kills bacteria and most viruses and is accomplished by using a tuberculocidal disinfectant. Dilute 1 part bleach in 100 parts water.

High-level disinfection is meant for use on medical devices and not environmental surfaces. It kills large numbers of pathogens, but does not completely eliminate them. Bacterial spores are left behind after disinfection. High-level disinfection uses heat pasteurization or a chemical disinfectant with a contact time of 12-45 minutes.

Low-level disinfection kills most bacteria and is accomplished by the use of general disinfectants. Antiseptics are designed for skin use. Do not use antiseptics on medical equipment or environmental surfaces.

DISINFECTION OF THE DIALYSIS FACILITY

Dialyzer facilities have regulations concerning the sterilization of the dialyzer and hemodialysis machine. Sterilization of these units is meant to control contamination by bacteria. It is typically recommended by the manufacturer that sodium hypochlorite be used on a regular basis and that a sterilant be used overnight at regular intervals. The concentration of sodium hypochlorite used in sterilization ranges from 500-5000 ppm. This translates to a dilution of 1:100 and 1:10 respectively.

After each patient, the equipment and furniture used should be wiped down with a bleach solution in a concentration between 1:100 and 1:10. Sterilization of the walls and floor is not necessary. Blood spills must be cleaned up at once. Contaminated linens and clothing should be put into a leak-proof bag for transport.

CDC RECOMMENDATIONS FOR CLEANING THE DIALYSIS MACHINE BETWEEN PATIENTS

CDC's recommendations for cleaning dialysis machines between patients:

- External transducer filters should be changed between patient treatments.
- Chairs, beds, dialysis machine, and tables should be cleaned and disinfected between patients.
- Give extra special attention to the cleaning of machine controls and front panels. These areas are frequently touched and can be contaminated even if they are not visibly dirty.
- Discard all fluids associated with dialyzer priming.
- Clean and disinfect receptacles between each patient.
- Never drape or clip bloodlines to a priming bucket or receptacle.
- Any visible soiling with blood or other matter should first be removed with a hospital grade germicidal detergent.
- Blood, mucous, or other debris can offer protection to microorganisms that are present and shield them from being destroyed in the disinfection process.
- After removing soil, clean the surfaces again with a general-purpose disinfectant.

CHEMICAL DISINFECTANTS

Chemical disinfectants are often used to sterilize the dialyzer. Renalin is the most commonly used chemical disinfectant. Formaldehyde is the second most commonly used disinfectant. Renalin is composed of hydrogen peroxide, peracetic acid, and acetic acid. To sterilize a dialyzer, a 0.5% solution of Renalin is used over an 11-hour time period. Aqueous formaldehyde kills spores and viruses as well as other microorganisms. A 4% concentration of aqueous formaldehyde can be used to sterilize a dialyzer and must be in contact with the unit for a minimum of 24 hours at room temperature. A dialyzer can also be sterilized using a 1.5% concentration of formalin at a temperature of 100 °F over a period of 24 hours.

HANDLING CHEMICAL DISINFECTANTS

Anyone sterilizing dialyzers with chemical disinfectants must wear appropriate protective gear. This includes an eye shield, waterproof gloves, and a waterproof gown. The Occupational Safety and Health Administration (OHSA) developed regulations for the use of hazardous chemicals, and these regulations must be posted. OSHA guidelines require adequate ventilation during the use of chemical disinfectants. If the chemical in use is splashed on the skin or in the eyes, the affected area should be flushed with large amounts of water. Medical advice and/or care should be sought. The staff handling the chemicals must be trained in their use and records of training must be kept. Safety Data Sheets (SDSs) outlining the methods to be used in handling the chemicals and the hazards associated with the chemicals must be posted.

HANDLING FORMALDEHYDE

The Occupational Safety and Health Administration (OSHA) regulations protect workers who may come in contact with formaldehyde. Formaldehyde is a suspected carcinogen. It is associated with the development of cancer of the lungs and nasal passages. Exposure through the air to as little as 0.1 ppm may result in irritation of the nasal passages, eyes, and throat. Exposure to this chemical may cause allergy- or asthma-like symptoms. These symptoms may include coughing or respiratory distress. Air quality is monitored where formaldehyde is in use. Permissible limits of exposure have been set by OSHA. All staff using formaldehyde must be trained in its use annually. An emergency shower and eyewash station must be readily available in case of accidents.

RECORDING MACHINE DISINFECTION

The recording of machine disinfection must be accurate and up-to-date as part of infection control to ensure that a contaminated machine is not in use and to verify that proper disinfection procedures were carried out. Disinfection procedures must follow manufacturers' guidelines and may vary somewhat. Elements to include in the disinfection record usually include:

- Date and time the process is initiated.
- Type of disinfection: Routine, monthly, complete system.
- Machine number or serial number.
- Cleaning of exterior machine: Disinfectant used.
- Type of internal disinfection process:
  - Rinse: Normal saline rinse.
  - Chlorine-based disinfectant: Disinfects and inhibits generation of calcium carbonate.
  - Peracetic acid-based: Contain peracetic and acetic acid and hydrogen peroxide to disinfect and dissolve calcium carbonate.
  - Acetic acid: Used to dissolve calcium carbonate deposits.
  - Formaldehyde: Disinfects but requires the technician to wear a respirator.
  - Citric/Malic acid: Used to dissolve calcium carbonate deposits.
  - Heat: >80 °C for 30 minutes.
- Note the concentration of chemicals used, along with dwell time, temperature, and duration for heat disinfection.
- Note the time the process is completed and signature or initials.

EMERGENCY EQUIPMENT

Emergency equipment that should be available on the dialysis unit includes:

- **Oxygen**: This may be available centrally or through tanks or oxygen concentrators. Full, partially used, and empty tanks must be kept separately and labeled. Pressure should be checked on the tanks when the regulator is attached and periodically during use to ensure the pressure doesn't fall below 200 psi. Batteries for concentrators should be checked on a regular basis. Central oxygen supply should be assessed routinely and backup oxygen supply available.

- **Crash cart**: All medications and supplies should be checked at least weekly and after each use to ensure supplies are all available according to the checklist and are intact and not expired.
- **AED**: Batteries should be checked on a routine schedule (weekly or monthly) and dates checked on AED pads to ensure they are not expired, which may cause them to fail to adhere properly. The defibrillator should be checked to ensure that it is functioning properly and that the cables are intact and secure.

ANCILLARY EQUIPMENT

Ancillary equipment on the dialysis unit includes:

- **pH meter**: Used to test the pH of dialysate. The electrode is placed in the solution and a small voltage released, and the voltage converted by the meter to a pH reading. To calibrate the meter, a test fluid with a specified pH should be tested to ensure that the pH readings are correct. For example, white vinegar has a pH of 2.9.
- **Multi-purpose digital dialysate meter**: Used to test for conductivity, total dissolved solids (TDS), oxidation reduction potential (ORD), pH, resistivity, and temperature and can be used to test both dialysate and water quality. A small sample of dialysate or other solution is placed in a sample cup on the meter. A sample with known values is used to calibrate the meter, but calibration must be done separately for different solution types. Calibration for the conductivity and pH of dialysate should be done at least at the beginning and end of each work day.

HEPARIN PUMP AND THE SINGLE-NEEDLE DEVICE

Heparin prevents blood from coagulating. Heparin is infused by means of a pump during dialysis to prevent the extracorporeal blood from clotting. There is an alarm system on the heparin pump to warn when the syringe containing the heparin is empty. The heparin pump can infuse at different rates as needed. The same pump can be used to infuse the venous line with protamine sulfate when regional heparinization is required.

Although two accesses are typically used in dialysis treatment, a single needle may be used. The **single-needle method** is not as efficient as the 2-needle method due to blood recirculation. If only one access is possible, the single-needle device is very useful. It permits the circulation of both arterial and venous blood at equal intervals at a maximum of about 300 mL/min.

RECOGNIZING ERRORS IN THE BLOOD AND DIALYSATE FLOW RATES

The blood flow rate and dialysate flow rate are programmed into the dialysis machines during the set up for the patient's treatment. The blood flow rate is usually about 300-500 L/min and dialysate rate is higher, at 300-1000 L/min. Alarms generally sound when flow rates are outside of the preset parameters, and this may indicate pump failure, blockage in a line, disconnection of a line, or (for dialysate) a low water pressure. If the settings are in error for the particular patient, then urea and fluid clearance may be inadequate. The clearance rate (urea removal) is related to the blood flow rate and the dialysate flow rate. If the clearance rate is too low, then increasing the blood flow rate may improve clearance, although the blood flow rate is limited to that tolerated by the fistula or graft. Increasing the dialysate flow rate may also improve clearance, but the amount of extra clearance beyond 600 mL/min is minimal. Extending the time of the treatment and/or utilizing a dialyzer with a larger surface area or clearance rating may also improve clearance.

RESISTANCE IN THE BLOOD CIRCUIT

The two main factors affecting resistance in the blood circuit are the viscosity (thickness) of the blood and the characteristics of the blood pathway. The viscosity of blood depends on the hematocrit. The characteristics of the blood pathway that affect resistance include the length, number of pathways, and the cross-sectional area. Low resistance is associated with short pathways. Lower resistance is found when there are a number of pathways. This is due to the division of resistance between pathways. A pathway with a large cross-section has low resistance. Hollow-fiber dialyzers have low resistance because of their short pathway, and large number of pathways. There are thousands of pathways with a hollow-fiber dialyzer. The internal radius of the fiber is the control factor for the hollow-fiber dialyzer.

Set-Up the Machine

PREPARING DIALYSIS EQUIPMENT FOR TREATMENT
PERFORMING RINSE PROCEDURES AND RESIDUAL CHEMICAL CHECKS

Preprocessing dialyzers before first use may wash out chemicals present in the manufacturing process. Once the dialyzer has been used and reprocessed, it must be rinsed thoroughly and checked for residual chemicals:

- Prime the arterial line prior to connecting it to the dialyzer.
- Rotate the dialyzer during the rinsing procedure to ensure that air pockets do not trap chemicals.
- Clamp the heparin line and make sure rinsing solution does not back up into the saline bag.
- Rinse the dialyzer thoroughly before sampling to check for chemicals.
- Replace the saline prime.
- Test the dialysis circuit with test strips for residual chemicals

After completion of the disinfection cycle for the dialysis machine and dialyzer, the rinsing solution is assessed for **residual chemicals** through rapid screening to determine if further rinsing is indicated:

- Residual chlorine test strip: Should be less than 0.1 ppm
- Residual peroxide test strip: Should be less than 3 ppm
- Formaldehyde test strip: Should be less than 3 ppm

PRIMING THE DIALYZER

It takes 500-1000 mL of normal saline to prime a dialyzer. The volume of fluid needed depends on the type and previous utilization of the dialyzer. Because the manufacturing process can leave glycerin and materials of various kinds in the dialyzer, it takes approximately 1000 mL of normal saline to prime a new dialyzer. It takes approximately 500 mL of normal saline to prime a reprocessed dialyzer.

Reprocessed dialyzers are filled with disinfectant. All disinfectant must be removed. No air should be allowed into the dialyzer. Air should be removed from the arterial bloodline by the infusion of saline prior to attaching the line to the dialyzer. After the arterial line is attached to the dialyzer, the unit should be turned so that the venous end is up. Priming is then continued.

ADDITIONAL STEPS FOR PREPARING THE DIALYZER

It is vitally important that all **air be removed** from the dialyzer. Trapped air could move across the dialysis membrane and into the patient's bloodstream. Air in the dialyzer decreases the efficiency of dialysis by preventing proper contact between the blood and dialysate and enhances the chances of dialyzer clotting. **Adequate flushing** with sterile normal saline solution serves to remove air and any particulate matter that may be present. Flushing also removes sterilant in reprocessing, making the dialyzer safe for contact with the patient's blood. The technician primes the dialyzer with the venous end up to push air pockets from the hollow fibers. The technician taps and rotates the dialyzer during priming to release air trapped in the headers.

PREPARING AUXILIARY EQUIPMENT

Auxiliary equipment that may be utilized during dialysis includes:

- **Oxygen**: Equipment, such as oxygen supply, tubing, nebulizer, and mask or nasal cannulas, should be readily available in an adequate supply. Depending on the oxygen source (tanks, central), the supply of oxygen should be verified daily.
- **Glucometer**: The glucometer's lens should be cleansed after each use and batteries checked on routine schedule and the glucometer calibrated as indicated according to manufacturer's recommendation (such as with a test strip when opening a new container of strips).
- **Conductivity meter**: The conductivity meter is built-in to the dialysis circuit for most machines and should show a display of the conductivity in millisiemens per centimeter (mS/cm). The conductivity cells (generally located both before and after the dialyzer) should be calibrated with an external meter by indicating the concentrate used, connecting the concentrate connectors to the concentrate solutions, connecting the dialysate lines to the external meter, recording values and comparing to the internal meter, and adjusting the internal meter as necessary. Conductivity settings should always be adjusted before the dialysis machine is in use, not during use.

ROTATING DIALYSIS EQUIPMENT IN THE DIALYSIS UNIT

It's important to rotate dialysis equipment. All available machines should be numbered sequentially and used in strict rotation to ensure so that all equipment is routinely in use and functioning correctly. In the event of an emergency situation (such as malfunction of a machine), the standby machines should be immediately available for use without the need for disinfection. Any dialysis machine that is not in use for more than 48 hours must be disinfected and rinsed prior to use and no more than 24 hours may elapse between disinfection and use, so maintaining equipment on standby and not using the equipment can result in the need for repeated disinfection procedures at additional cost to the dialysis center in terms of chemical disinfectants and staff time needed to disinfect. Equipment supplies (needles, tubing, concentrates) should also be rotated so that the oldest supplies and equipment are always used first in order to avoid unnecessary waste from having to dispose of or reprocess those that are outdated.

REQUIRED SAFETY CHECKS ON THE DIALYSIS MACHINE

PH AND CONDUCTIVITY

Safety checks on the dialysis machine include:

- **pH**: The dialysate should be checked before each use to ensure that the pH is in the recommended range of 6.8-7.6. The pH may be monitored with an external digital dialysate meter, test strips, or (with some models) by the internal meter included in the machine. Additionally, the water used in the system should be routinely checked for pH and corrected if needed as water is sometimes too alkaline for adequate removal of contaminants.

- **Conductivity**: This meter is used to check the proportioning system, which dilutes the concentrates (electrolytes) with incoming water to produce the appropriate dialysate. The meter continuously monitors the dilution and shows the degree of conductivity, which reflects the concentration of electrolytes. Normal values range from 12-16 mS/cm. When the range falls outside these parameters, alarms sound and can indicate that the concentration has changed, water pressure is abnormal, leaks have occurred in the mixing chamber, the system has a fault, such as a disconnected line, or a concentration jug is empty. When alarms sound, the system automatically reroutes the dialysate to a drain to protect the patient.

TEMPERATURE

The **dialysate heater** is controlled by one or more electronic regulators that are designed to keep the dialysate temperature at asset rate within 0.5 °C of the set point. Machines are equipped with sensors that continuously monitor the temperature and create an alarm if the dialysate exceeds a safe limit. Many patients on dialysis have a lower body temperature than the general population, so if dialysate temperature is set too high, it causes vasodilatation, leading to increased hypotension and inability of the blood vessels to counter-regulate due to volume expansion. Dialysate temperatures over 41 °C can cause the rupture (hemolysis) of red blood cells, which continues past the end of dialysis.

ADDITIONAL ELEMENTS OF THE PRE-ASSESSMENT OF THE DIALYZER

The dialyzer must be checked to ensure that it is functioning properly prior to the initiation of treatment. Elements of the pre-assessment of the dialyzer include:

- The integrity of the dialyzer membrane must be ensured.
- The bloodlines should be checked to ensure that there are no leaks or kinks.
- It must be determined that the dialysate prescription is correct and that the composition correctly reflects the prescription.
- The potassium and calcium levels of the dialysate must be checked to ensure that they are correct.
- The temperature of the dialysate must be taken to determine if they are in the range of 35-37 °C.
- The dialysis delivery system must be determined to be free of sterilant or disinfectant.
- The circuit must be determined to be free of air.
- The blood pump must be occluded properly.
- The tubing must be seated properly.
- The alarms must be set.
- The water to be used for dialysis must be checked for chloramines.

TESTING ALARMS
CHECKING ALARMS PRIOR TO INITIATION OF TREATMENT

The **alarms** on the dialyzer must be checked to ensure that they are working properly. Malfunctioning alarms may cause the dialyzer to stop functioning and interfere with treatment. For example, if the arterial or venous pressure alarms are triggered when they shouldn't be, the blood pump will stop and the venous line will close. An alarm that is not triggered when something is wrong can cause harm to the patient.

DIALYSIS FLOW METERS AND PRESSURE MONITORS

The accumulation of solute film can reduce the accuracy of the flow meter. The accuracy of the flow meter must be monitored and the flow meter must be calibrated as a regular part of maintenance. Flow rate can be determined by collecting outflow from the drain hose and measuring the volume of fluid collected in a certain period of time.

Ultrafiltration may be controlled by adjusting the negative pressure of the dialysate. In this case, it is necessary that **inflow and outflow monitors have set points for high and low pressure**. An alarm should sound when pressure gets too high or too low. The set points of this alarm must be accurate to within 20 mmHg above or below, or 10% of the reading. The manufacturer provides directions regarding the calibration of the monitors. Ultrafiltration may also be controlled volumetrically or flowmetrically. In this scenario, pressure monitors serve to monitor the transmembrane pressure.

ONLINE CLEARANCE MONITORING

Online clearance monitoring is a noninvasive method used to **measure the level of clearance during a dialysis treatment**. Sodium chloride is used as a marker for urea because it has a similar molecular weight (58 and 60 respectively). The program tests clearance in 2 stages. First, the sodium concentration in the dialysate is raised above the concentration in the blood to as much as 15.5 mS/cm for 2-3 minutes. This increase in the dialysis sodium causes the sodium to cross the membrane and enter the blood through the process of diffusion. The second stage of the test involves decreasing the sodium concentration of the dialysate to 13.5 mS/cm, which causes the sodium to cross the membrane. A clearance value is calculated by taking the difference between the conductivity of the fluid at the inlet and outlet flow paths. The removal of urea from the blood can be predicted from this value.

VENOUS PRESSURE

Venous pressure is a measurement of the pressure in the corporeal blood circuit after the blood exits the dialyzer, but before it enters the patient's body again. Venous pressure is a measurement of the resistance of the blood re-entering the patient's vascular system by way of the venous needle. The line used to monitor this pressure is connected to the upper part of the venous bubble trap. A marked and rapid increase in venous pressure may indicate a kinked venous line, a clot in the bubble trap, a clot in the venous needle, a misplaced venous needle, or a failing vascular access. A decrease in venous pressure may indicate a displaced venous needle, a wet transducer, or a clot in the arterial chamber.

ARTERIAL PRESSURE

Arterial pressure in this context is not a measurement of the patient's systemic arterial blood pressure. It is a measurement of the pressure in the extracorporeal blood circuit that runs between the site of insertion of the arterial needle and a location proximal to the blood pump. The blood pump creates negative pressure, of which arterial pressure is actually a measurement. Excess suction on the vascular access can be prevented by monitoring arterial pressure. A sudden increase in arterial pressure could indicate that the needle is clotted or displaced. It could also indicate that the arterial line has a kink or that the patient's systemic blood pressure has dropped. A change in the arterial negative pressure will trigger the alarm and turn off the blood pump. A high negative arterial pressure may cause damage to the vascular access. Furthermore, it may result in hemolysis of the red blood cells.

BLOOD LEAK DETECTOR

The effluent dialysis line contains detectors that check for blood leaks. The detector consists of a beam of light and a photocell. The light is shone through the dialysate and received by the photocell. Any change in the translucence and light scatter of the dialysis fluid activates the alarms and stops the dialysis process. Standards established by the AAMI require that the test be sensitive enough to detect a change of less than 0.35-0.45 mL/min of blood (depending on the type of alarm) at hematocrit 25%. The criterion applies to a range of dialysis fluid flows. False alarms may be caused by air bubbles and particles in the fluid. If the alarm sounds and the blood leak cannot be seen, a Hemastix should be used to check for a leak.

AIR BUBBLE DETECTORS

Air bubble detectors are situated in the venous bubble trap. They work by passing a sonic beam through the chamber. Sound travels quicker through fluid than through air, so when the air bubble detector beam is interrupted by the presence of foam or even tiny air bubbles, it triggers a clamp that shuts of the venous blood flow to the patient and stops the blood pump. The technician must correct the cause and reset the alarm manually before dialysis can begin again. Air can come from loose connections; cracked tubing, connectors, or portions of the dialyzer; and from fluid bags connected to the dialysate circuit. Since infusing an air embolus into a patient may be fatal, never place a patient on a machine with a disarmed air detector even for a second. It is too easy to forget it is disarmed and walk away, perhaps costing the patient's life.

PROCEDURE FOR CHECKING THE DIALYZER FOR AIR AND FLUSHING THE DIALYZER

Any air present in the dialyzer must be flushed out. Air from the dialyzer could jeopardize patient health by allowing air to pass through the membrane into the patient's vascular system. Air in the dialyzer unit will reduce the efficiency of the dialyzer. The air will interfere with clearance by preventing diffusion between the blood and dialysate. If the dialyzer is of the hollow-fiber type, air can get trapped in the fibers and cause clotting. The dialyzer must be primed with saline to flush out any particles left over from the manufacturing process. The dialyzer must be free of any residual disinfectant. Physiologic saline should be used to flush and prime the dialyzer. Physiologic saline is composed of 0.9 g NaCl per 100 mL water. Physiologic saline is used because it is compatible with blood.

CONSEQUENCES OF AIR IN THE DIALYZER

The functioning of the dialyzer creates negative pressure at the intake side. Because of this negative pressure, air can be sucked into the dialyzer. Air can enter the dialyzer at a number of points. Ill-fitting connections can allow air to enter the system. For example, if the connection at the needle hub is not tight enough, air can enter at this point. Needle punctures and holes in the tubing can result in air entering the system. Empty fluid containers can also be the source of unwanted air in the dialyzer. Air in the dialyzer interferes with its functioning and safety. The hollow fibers of the hollow-fiber artificial kidney can become blocked by air in the blood. Air in the system passing through the venous bubble trap can result in the patient suffering an air embolism.

DETECTION OF AIR, FOAM, AND MICROBUBBLES

An **ultrasonic beam** is often used to detect air, foam, and microbubbles in the blood in the dialyzer. This system works on the principle that sound waves travel through fluid faster than they travel through air. If the sound waves meet a bubble, they slow down and an alarm is set off. Air/foam detectors do not usually have a method to adjust the sensitivity externally. A saline solution will not set off the alarm and conditions in the surrounding environment will not set off the alarm. During maintenance procedures, such as priming and rinsing, the alarm system can be disarmed. The dialysis unit should never be used on a patient when the air/foam detector is disarmed.

DIALYSATE

The dialysis fluid, or dialysate, serves to carry away the waste products and fluid that the dialysis procedure has removed from the blood. The dialysis fluid also prevents the loss of necessary electrolytes and the loss of excess fluid during the dialysis treatment. The chemical composition of the dialysis fluid is designed to match that of normal plasma water as closely as possible. Dialysate is usually composed of five compounds: sodium chloride (NaCl), sodium bicarbonate ($NaHCO_3$), chloride, calcium, potassium, and magnesium. In addition, some dialysate formulas include glucose. Dialysis concentrate is available commercially in containers of several sizes. The concentrate may also be made on site from dry chemicals. Making the dialysate on site can save in transportation costs.

CHECKING DIALYSATE COMPOSITION

Primary methods of testing the dialysate composition include laboratory tests to measure the concentration of a particular solute. The concentrations of two solutes are typically determined. For example, the concentration of sodium can be measured by flame photometry. The concentration of chloride can be measured by titration.

Total conductivity is a secondary test used to assess dialysate concentration. It measures the total conductivity contributed by the total number of ions. Conductivity is measured by a meter that must be calibrated. There is a safe range for each type of concentrate. The conductivity of the concentrate when it is mixed properly is usually indicated on the label of the container. Another secondary check of the composition of the dialysate is the total osmolality. This is tested by freezing point depression or vapor pressure. These are used to measure total solute.

ACHIEVEMENT OF ACID-BASE BALANCE IN DIALYSIS

Two types of concentrates are used in dialysis. These are an **acid concentrate** and a **bicarbonate concentrate**. The bicarbonate concentrate contains sodium bicarbonate and sodium chloride. The sodium chloride increases conductivity and allows monitoring. The acid concentrate and bicarbonate concentrate are blended in the appropriate proportions with water.

The inclusion of bicarbonate in the dialysate is necessary with the use of short, rapid dialysis and high-flux dialysis. Bicarbonate is used in dialysis to treat the acidosis that occurs with renal failure. The dialysis treatment involves the transfer of bicarbonate from the dialysate compartment to the blood compartment. The bicarbonate buffers the hydrogen ions and helps the body to reach an acid-base balance.

The pH of the dialysis fluid must be monitored. Normally the pH level should be within the range of 6.8-7.6. If the pH is found to be outside of these limits, an alarm system should sound. The alarm system should include visual and audile signals. The pH sensors must be recalibrated on a regular basis as they tend to drift.

DIALYSATE TEMPERATURE

It is necessary to regulate the temperature of the dialysate. This is accomplished with the use of a heater, a heat exchanger, or both. The temperature of the dialysis fluid should be kept within 0.5 °C of the set point. The temperature of the dialysis fluid should be monitored on a continuing basis with a sensor that operates independently of the heat control. Visible and audible alarms should sound if the temperature strays from desirable limits. The accuracy of the heat sensor should be tested with a glass thermometer on a regular basis in case of malfunctions. Patients with end-stage renal disease often have a core temperature of 36.0-36.5 °C. Excessively warm dialysis fluid can cause vasodilation at a time when the body is undergoing vasoconstriction to minimize hypotension. If the dialysis fluid temperature exceeds 41 °C, hemolysis of the red blood cells can occur.

IMPACT OF AERATION ON DIALYSATE TEMPERATURE

Dissolved air and **microbubbles** are found in water in substantial amounts. The air that is dissolved in the water forms microbubbles as the water is warmed. These microbubbles adversely affect dialysate temperature and interfere with the functioning of conductivity sensors and flow meters. In addition, the bubbles formed when the fluid heats up can reduce the contact of the dialysate with the dialysis membrane in hollow-fiber dialyzers. The dissolved air must be removed from the solution and this is done by means of warmers and negative pressure. The freed gases are then trapped in an air trap and directed to the outside where they can't interfere with the functioning of the dialyzer.

ISSUES AND PROTOCOLS REGARDING CONTAMINANTS IN DIALYSATE

The Association for the Advancement of Medical Instrumentation (AAMI) has established standards for allowable contaminants in dialysate. The standards regarding bacteria are expressed in terms of total viable count (TVC) of bacteria (CFU). The minimum regulatory requirement states that there can be no more than 100 TVC bacteria per milliliter in water used for dialysis. In addition, there can be no more than 100 CFU bacteria as measured by the LAL test in the dialysis fluid exiting the delivery system. This measurement can also be expressed as 0.25 EU/mL (the AAMI's minimum regulatory standard). Bacteria multiply in the dialysis fluid as it moves through the dialyzer. As a result of reverse filtration, pyrogenic materials cross the membrane into the blood. A molecular or ultrafilter can be placed in the dialysate pathway in front of the dialyzer. A 50,000- to 100,000-Da ultrafilter can screen out intact endotoxins while a 1000- to 10,000-Da ultrafilter is needed to screen out fragments.

MAKING BICARBONATE-BASED DIALYSATE

Calcium and magnesium do not form a stable solution when mixed with bicarbonate. This is due to the low hydrogen ion content. For this reason, when making bicarbonate-based dialysate, two separate concentrates must be used. The dialysate delivery system must then be more complex to prepare and regulate 3 liquids instead of only 2 liquids. The chemicals contained in the 2 concentrates used in bicarbonate-based dialysate are as follows. The chemicals in the A (acidified) concentrate include sodium, calcium, magnesium, potassium, chloride, and acetic acid. The acetic acid serves to maintain a low pH so that the calcium and magnesium stays in the solution. The B (bicarbonate) concentrate is composed of sodium bicarbonate and sometimes some sodium chloride.

MIXING AND VERIFYING BICARBONATE SOLUTIONS

Bicarbonate neutralizes acids, which tend to build up in the blood, causing a low pH between dialysis treatments. The normal range of bicarbonate is 22-26 mEq/L. In order to ensure that bicarbonate diffuses into the blood during dialysis in order to reduce acids, the bicarbonate level must be set slightly higher than the level in the blood. Procedures for mixing and verifying bicarbonate solution (which may also contain sodium) vary according to the type of system and the size of the tank (and some systems use cartridges that do not require manual mixing or individual jugs), but general procedures include:

- Ensuring that the tank is empty and has been cleaned and disinfected before beginning.
- Closing all values and checking switches to make sure they are turned off.
- Filling the tank according to manufacturer's instructions.
- Turning on the mixer.

- Opening the lid and adding the dry bicarbonate powder or liquid according to the desired proportion.
- Mixing for the prescribed period of time (such as 10 minutes) to ensure the bicarbonate is completely dissolved.
- Obtaining a sample from a valve at the base of the tank and checking bicarbonate level.

DISADVANTAGES OF BICARBONATE SOLUTIONS

Disadvantages of bicarbonate dialysate include the following:

- Bicarbonate concentrate is **unstable in liquid form**. A polymer may be added by the manufacturer to stabilize the concentrate. Dry sodium bicarbonate ($NaHCO_4$) may be provided by the manufacturer so that the powder can be mixed at the facility. The resulting solution must be used within 24 hours.
- Bicarbonate concentrate is **very easily contaminated** by bacteria. The stabilized bicarbonate solution is also easily contaminated and should not be used if the container holding it has been opened for more than 72 hours. It is necessary to sanitize all containers that are used in the preparation, storage, and dispensing of B concentrate on a continual basis. The A concentrate comes in many formulations to allow variations in dialysis prescription. As each dialysate delivery system is unique in its proportioning and mixing ratios, care must be taken to select the correct concentrates for the system.

MIXING ACID SOLUTIONS

The acid concentrate (also referred to as the **electrolyte solution**) added to water to produce dialysate contains specific amounts of the electrolytes, such as potassium, sodium, magnesium, and calcium, as well as glucose. The acidifier decreases the dialysate's pH. The acidifier should be added to the system before the bicarbonate in order to prevent the formation of calcium carbonate precipitates. Before adding the concentrate, the contents should be examined to ensure there is a sufficient amount for the entire treatment(s) because running out in the middle of the treatment will result in problems with conductivity. The acid (usually red) connector is connected to the acid jug (for individual treatment) or the centralized acid supply (when the same solution is used for multiple patients). The hemodialysis technician should then check the displays and verify that the concentration type matches that prescribed. Once the concentrations are verified, most machines require that the values be confirmed. Proportioning systems that control the mixing and correct proportion of concentrate to water are built into the dialysis machines.

PROPORTIONING SYSTEM

A proportioning system is used to mix the proper proportions of liquid concentrates. Microprocessor circuitry is often used to regulate the speed of the pump. The fluid is monitored downstream to ensure that the proportions are correct. There is an electronic feedback system to control the speed of the pump and the volumes of concentrates that go into the mixture.

Proportioning systems are complex and expensive. They are both electronic and hydraulic. Many of the functions of proportioning systems are preprogrammed and are not easily changeable. It is often difficult to find the cause of any problem. Redundant systems are necessary. Personnel from the factory are often needed to repair the system in the event of a system breakdown.

CONTROL OF DIALYSATE CONCENTRATION WITH THE PROPORTIONING UNIT

The proportioning unit ensures that the correct proportions of treated water and concentrate are mixed. This **proportion is 34:1.** The proportioning unit has a built-in conductivity meter to monitor the concentration of the dialysate. The meter must be temperature-compensated. The accuracy of the meter is 1-3% above or below normal. If the concentration of the dialysate changes, then the flow of the dialysate will be redirected. This ensures that the patient does not receive dialysate of the wrong concentration. An alarm also sounds when the dialysate concentration is incorrect. Most dialyzer systems use two conductivity meters and the readings on these must match. If the conductivity meters show an incorrect dialysate concentration, laboratory tests should be conducted to check the concentration.

DIALYSATE DELIVERY SYSTEMS

The dialysate delivery system prepares the dialysis fluid and sends it to the dialyzer unit. Dialysate delivery systems may deliver dialysis fluid to one dialyzer station or to several stations at the same time. The solution delivery system (SDS) is designed to transport the solutions needed to prepare the dialysis fluid to the dialyzer unit. The bicarbonate and acid needed to make the dialysis fluid are transferred from a mixing tank and storage tank respectively to an overhead holding tank. This holding tank is called a head tank. The resulting solution is directed through a solution distribution system and then sent to the patient care area. From the patient care area, the solution is fed to the dialyzer unit through a series of pipes.

SORBENT REGENERATIVE SUPPLY SYSTEM

The sorbent regenerative supply system recirculates the dialysate through a cartridge containing adsorbent material. In this way, the dialysate is regenerated chemically. The dialysate is cleansed of waste products and the electrolytes and pH restored to desired levels. The sorbent regenerative supply system cleans the dialysate in a number of ways. Urea is converted to ammonia carbonate. Creatinine and other nonionized particles in the dialysate are adsorbed. Ion-exchange resins are utilized. The cartridge of the system is divided into segments.

The dialysis fluid flows into the **first segment** of the cartridge of the sorbent regenerative supply system and passes through a *carbon layer*. The carbon layer removes the heavy metal and oxidants from the dialysate. The dialysis fluid then flows into a section of the cartridge containing an enzyme called *urease* that breaks down urea. The urease converts the urea to ammonium and carbonate.

The dialysate continues to flow into the **second segment** of the cartridge, which contains *sodium zirconium phosphate*. This substance behaves as an exchange resin. It absorbs the ammonium ions and releases sodium and hydrogen ions in a ratio of 1 Na+ to 9 H+. The carbonate ion and hydrogen ions interact to form bicarbonate ions and carbon dioxide. The sodium zirconium phosphate in the cartridge exchanges calcium, magnesium, and potassium ions for sodium ions.

The **third segment** of the cartridge, which contains *hydrated zirconium oxide*, clears phosphate ions and fluoride from the dialysate.

The **fourth and last segment** of the cartridge contains *activated carbon* (charcoal). The activated carbon adsorbs creatinine, uric acid, guanidine, and other metabolites of organic origin contained in the dialysate.

It is necessary to infuse the dialysate with some ions before the fluid is returned to the dialyzer. Calcium and magnesium are replaced, and potassium may be added.

ADVANTAGES AND DISADVANTAGES

There are distinct advantages to the sorbent regenerative supply system. The system is portable and only needs a source of electricity. There is no need for a supply of special water, and drains are not necessary.

There are also disadvantages to using this system. The sorbent regenerative supply system is expensive, and the cartridges are costly. The system has limitations. It can only process a certain amount of urea and ammonia. The system may not be able to absorb all the ammonia, resulting in buildup in not only the system but also in the patient's blood. More than one cartridge may be required to treat large patients. In addition, more than one cartridge may be needed if the patient has a very high serum urea level.

CONFIRMATION OF RECIRCULATION CONCENTRATION

Any substance in the arterial bloodline entering the dialyzer should be in the same concentration as it is in the systemic circulation of the patient. If the concentration of a substance is lower in the arterial bloodline, it may be due to dilution. The venous blood returning from the dialyzer may be entering the arterial bloodline and diluting the substance. An estimate of the recirculation can be calculated from 3 blood samples. One sample is from the systemic (peripheral) circulation. This is sample P. A second sample (sample A) is taken from the arterial blood in the inflow line before the blood enters the dialyzer. The third sample (sample V) is taken from the venous blood in the outflow line after it leaves the dialyzer. The estimated recirculation is calculated as follows: (P-A) divided by (P-V). Recirculation should not be more than 5-10%.

DOCUMENTING IN DAILY EQUIPMENT LOGS

Equipment logs must be kept up-to-date and accurate in order to meet regulatory requirements and to ensure the safety of the equipment in order to prevent patient complications/injuries. Equipment logs may include:

- **Reprocessing log**: From the date of receipt until the dialyzer is disposed of, every step in processing and reprocessing must be recorded.
- **Dialyzer problem log**: Record the date and time of any problems encountered for specific dialyzers, such as blood leaks or impaired performance, and note any actions taken to correct the problem.
- **Environmental testing log**: Results of testing for cleaning agents in effluent and dialyzer rinse, including date, time, and type of testing.
- **Equipment maintenance log**: Dates, times, and results of all routine preventive maintenance and testing, and repairs.
- **Inventory logs**: Record of receipt of new equipment, quality control testing results, first use, and expiration dates.

Evaluate Machine Operation

DIALYZER REUSE

Dialyzers may be cleaned, sterilized, and prepared after use for reuse on the same patient. Dialyzer reuse is a common practice that helps to keep costs under control. Many clinics reuse dialyzers safely. There are advantages and disadvantages to dialyzer reuse. On the plus side, reusing dialyzers significantly reduces the average cost per dialysis treatment. When a dialyzer is used for the first time, it may produce the "first-use syndrome." This syndrome is uncommon but occurs occasionally with new cellulose dialyzers during the first half hour of a treatment. The symptoms include chest pain, back pain, nausea, and general discomfort. This syndrome does not occur with reused dialyzers. There are several disadvantages to the reuse of dialyzers. Getting the dialyzer ready for reuse is time-consuming and requires large amounts of high-quality water. The agents used in sterilization may pose a health hazard to patients and personnel.

CRITERIA

Dialyzer reuse was common practice in the late 1990's, but with increasing evidence of bloodstream infections resulting from dialyzer reuse, this practice is now used less frequently. Currently, in order to be approved for reuse, the dialyzer must be identified by the manufacturer as appropriate for reuse and then carefully reprocessed. Criteria for reprocessing are as follows:

- The dialyzer must be appropriately **rinsed** (most often with normal saline, but some facilities may use hydrogen peroxide) within 2 hours.
- The dialyzer must be **cleaned**. The most recommended and used cleaning agent is Renalin (consisting of peracetic acid). Bleach may be used in some centers.
- The dialyzer's **performance** must be tested.
  - It must have sufficient solute removal capacity remaining. This can be determined by a total cell volume (TCV) measurement. The unit is filled with water, and as much of this water as possible is pumped out. The volume of water pumped out is measured using a graduated cylinder. Per KDOQI guidelines, if the cylinder contains less than 80% of the original volume filling the dialyzer, the dialyzer cannot be reused. Urea clearance can also be measured, and cannot be below 90% of the dialyzer's original urea clearance.
  - The dialyzer is also pressure tested, or leak tested, to determine if there are any broken fibers within the membrane. Broken fibers can cause blood leaks during the dialysis treatment. The dialyzer cannot be reused if large streaks of blood can be seen. This indicates that there are a large number of clotted fibers.
  - The dialyzer's ultrafiltration coefficient must also be tested.

CONTRAINDICATIONS TO REUSING THE DIALYZER

While less common, reuse is a clinically and ethically accepted practice if proper precautions are taken. Reusing dialyzers is an economically and environmentally sound practice. However, it is important to note that it is not always medically appropriate to reuse a dialyzer. If the dialysis patient has a systemic infection or sepsis, he or she is usually not included in the reuse program. Dialysis patients with hepatitis B cannot be included in reprocessing programs. Reuse of the dialyzer is not permitted if the patient does not give written consent. This is a regulation of the Centers for Medicare and Medicaid Services (CMS). The written consent to allow the reuse of the dialyzer becomes part of the patient's medical record.

EQUIPMENT MAINTENANCE RECORDS

The equipment maintenance log should be maintained on site and must be kept up-to-date to ensure that all preventive maintenance is carried out and all equipment is safe to use and in running order. Additionally, the logs serve as evidence that regulatory requirements regarding maintenance have been completed. Most equipment logs have separates page or files for each equipment item so that the history of each piece of equipment can be easily accessed. Logs may require narrative explanations or use checklists. Elements of the equipment maintenance log vary from one facility to another but may include:

- Date, time, and signature.
- Type of equipment.
- Unit or serial number of the equipment.
- Due dates for routine preventive maintenance.
- Dates actual preventive maintenance carried out.
- Problems encountered in maintenance and actions taken.
- Repairs carried out.

- Type of testing carried out.
- Results of testing.

Water Treatment

Components/Design of Systems

DIALYSIS WATER TREATMENT

The dialysis membrane cannot filter out all the undesirable substances in water to be used for dialysis. There are a number of methods used to treat water to be used in dialysis. These include mechanical filtration, the use of water softeners (to reduce calcium and magnesium levels in the case of hard water), reverse osmosis, deionization, exposure to ultraviolet light, and filtration by activated carbon. Activated carbon cleanses water of substances by adsorption. Different treatment techniques are useful for removing different substances from the water. The Association for the Advancement of Medical Instrumentation (AAMI) has established guidelines in conjunction with the Organization for Standardization (ISO) and the American National Standards Institute (ANSI) regarding the quality of water used in dialysis. Standards have been developed that apply to both to inorganic and microbiologic contaminants. These guidelines are accepted as the standard in the United States. Local guidelines/standards may also apply.

Generally, a water treatment system should be used in dialysis centers that meets the local and federal regulations regarding dialysis water quality. A water treatment system usually consists of three parts: pretreatment, primary treatment (and possibly a secondary treatment), and distribution.

DIALYSIS WATER TREATMENT VS. DRINKING WATER TREATMENT

Many times, the amount of water that is ingested from drinking is far less than that which comes into contact with a hemodialysis patient's blood during a treatment. A substance in water may be safe at certain levels, but harmful at higher levels. For example, a substance may be safe for drinking as the substance is ingested at a safe level, but when the substance is in dialysis fluid, the patient may come into contact with amounts exceeding the safe level of the substance. In addition, the gastrointestinal tract processes the drinking water that is ingested before it reaches the bloodstream. The gastrointestinal tract can regulate the speed at which substances in the water are absorbed. In a patient on dialysis, substances pass through the dialysis membrane by diffusion and contact with the bloodstream is not controlled.

LAL TEST AND WATER USED TO PREPARE DIALYSATE

LAL stands for **limulus amebocyte lysate**. The LAL assay is an *in vitro* test used to detect and quantify endotoxin. The test uses a protein extract from the horseshoe crab. The results of the assay are expressed in nanograms per mL (ng/mL). The test can also be expressed in endotoxin units (EU). For comparison and conversion, 1 ng/mL equals 5 EU/mL.

Water used in dialysis must meet the standards set forth by the AAMI. These standards outline acceptable chemical, bacterial, and pyrogen content. Water used in the manufacturing of dialysate must have a microbial count lower than 200 total viable count (TVC)/mL per AAMI's minimum regulatory standard, with the preferred recommendation being a count of less than 100 TVC. The concentration of endotoxins in the water must be less than 2 EU/mL, with the preferred recommendation being a count of less than 0.25 EU. Various processes must be followed to ensure that the water used in the preparation of dialysis meets the required standards.

USE OF TAP WATER IN DIALYSIS

Tap water may contain impurities that can harm a patient on dialysis. These impurities include organic and inorganic chemicals and bacteria. The inorganic chemicals present in the water vary with the geographical region, as different inorganic chemicals are found in different locations. Tap water that has been deemed fit to drink is not necessarily safe to use in dialysis. Any contaminants found in the tap water may enter the dialysis patient's bloodstream. In addition, untreated tap water may have a pH that is too high or too low. Some delivery systems will not function if the water is too acidic or too alkaline. Dialysis fluid must be made from water of high purity.

SELECTING THE WATER PROCESSING SYSTEM

The type of water processing system chosen to prepare dialysis fluid depends on the solute content of the available tap water. **Feed water**, the water before the treatment process has started, should be analyzed regularly to monitor its chemical and bacteriologic content. Prior to treatment, the feed water should meet the Environmental Protection Agency (EPA) requirements for drinking water. The **product water**, the water after treatment, should meet the standards set by the AAMI. The product water is used to make the dialysate. Different treatments may be necessary to meet the requirements in different areas, depending upon the qualities of the feed water. Water treatment may include the following systems: initial sediment filter; resin-type softener; activated carbon filter; reverse osmosis (RO) module; and deionizing unit.

MECHANICAL FILTRATION OF DIALYSIS WATER

Mechanical filtration can remove particles suspended in the water. Suspended particles may include mud, rust, and algae. Mechanical filtration can be accomplished using a wound filament or a membrane cartilage. It can also be accomplished through the use of tanks holding granular material through which the water is filtered. This material can be backflushed. These methods can be used to filter out particles as small as 5 mm in size. Smaller particles of 0.2 mm can be filtered out using submicron filters. Different filters are capable of removing particles of different sizes from the water. Filters are numbered according to the size of the particles they can remove from a liquid. Filters with smaller numbers are capable of removing smaller particles from a liquid.

CARBON TANKS

The carbon tank works through the **process of adsorption**. Carbon tanks are able to cleanse the water of chlorines and chloramines. The adsorptive properties of the carbon tank also allow it to remove organic material from the water. The carbon tank can also cleanse the water of materials that cause odors. The process of adsorption involves the adherence of substances to a surface. In the case of the carbon tank, the surface to which the substances adhere is the activated carbon. The substances that can be filtered out by the carbon tank include liquids, gases, and suspended particles. Electrolytes cannot be removed from the water by use of an activated carbon filter.

UTILIZATION

Water treatment systems using carbon tanks usually use two such tanks. The first tank clears the water of almost all the chlorine. The second tank is used to back up the first tank in the event that not all the chlorine was removed. The first and second tanks may be called the working tank and the polishing tank, respectively. To ensure efficient adsorption, the tanks are backwashed. This redistributes the carbon in the tank. Because the polishing tank has little flow through it and therefore little chlorine running through it, bacteria may flourish in the tank. Either tank may be used as the working or polishing tank. The tanks may be rotated in order to extend the life of the tanks.

TYPES

There are two types of carbon tanks used to filter dialysis water. These are the portable exchange carbon tank and permanent portable exchange carbon tank.

- **Portable exchange tanks** are used for a period of time and then replaced. The cycle of use and replacement is set by the dialysis facility. The complete tank is replaced by the vendor.
- **Permanent portable tanks** are designed so that they can be backwashed. The facility decides the schedule for backwashing. Backwashing redistributes the carbon, and removes the channels in the carbon bed, but it does not regenerate the carbon. The redistribution of the carbon allows the entire carbon bed to come into contact with the water being filtered. The carbon is replaced by the vendor as necessary.

WATER SOFTENERS

The water softener is used in conjunction with the carbon tanks. It is placed after the carbon tanks to exchange ions in the water being treated. Water is considered hard because of its calcium and magnesium ion content. The purpose of the water softener is to replace calcium and magnesium ions with sodium ions. Ions are exchanged on the basis of mill equivalency (mEq). The water softener will also clear the water of other positive ions. Two sodium ions are added to the water for every calcium ion that is removed. The sodium is later cleared from the water by the process of reverse osmosis. Some types of water softeners have a concentrated brine tank attached. The purpose of the brine tank is to store the sodium chloride and to permit regeneration of the softener at the dialysis facility.

REVERSE OSMOSIS FOR WATER TREATMENT

Reverse osmosis (RO) is the most advanced system designed to treat water to be used in dialysis. The water is treated by other methods before RO is used. The RO removes the majority of contaminants that were not removed by the previous treatment or treatments. In RO, water under high pressure is pushed across a semipermeable membrane. The particles dissolved in the water are screened by the membrane and collect on the feed side. The pure water will continue through the membrane and collect on the other side. The RO system will screen out bacteria, viruses, and pyrogens. The filtered water is purified after RO. The purified water is then collected in a holding tank for later use.

CHARACTERISTICS AND TYPES OF MEMBRANES

Membranes used in RO must have certain **characteristics**:

- The membranes must allow water to pass through freely.
- The membranes must be able to screen out solutes. Therefore, they must be highly impermeable to dissolved particles.
- The membranes must be strong enough to stand up to high pressure.
- The ideal membrane can also tolerate widely varying pH levels and widely varying temperatures.
- The ideal membrane is resistant to the actions of bacteria and chemicals.

There are a number of types of membranes that can be used in RO. The membrane types commonly in use with RO include cellulose acetate membranes, polyamide membranes, thin-film composite membranes, and chlorine-resistant polysulfone membranes. These membranes all have different strengths and weaknesses.

CHLORINE AND AMMONIA AND THE USE OF A HOLDING TANK

Chlorine and ammonia are sometimes put into the city water supply to kill bacteria. The chemical reaction between chlorine and ammonia creates oxidant compounds called chloramines. Chloramines are nonionic and are not rejected by the RO membrane. Some dialysis patients have developed anemia as a result of exposure to chloramine. Chloramine can be removed from the water by the use of a carbon filter, and this should be done before running the water through an RO system.

Hemodialysis units often make use of a holding tank for processed water from the RO unit. The water is circulated in a loop between the RO unit and holding tank. Microbes and endotoxins may grow in the holding tank and the pipes. The tanks must be designed in such a way as to discourage their growth. Chlorine and iodine may be used to limit the growth of microbes and endotoxins.

ADVANTAGES

The reverse osmosis (RO) system has a number of advantages over other types of water treatments. The RO membrane prevents the passage of bacteria, viruses, pyrogens, and pyrogen fragments. The purity of water treated by RO is similar in composition to distilled water. Because the units are compact, they can be used at home. The units are relatively small and require little space to set up. The membrane usually has a useful life of 1-2 years. After this period of time, replacement is necessary. The length of time that the membrane lasts depends on the type of membrane being used. The entire system can be sterilized as required with formalin or with another type of sterilant.

DISADVANTAGES

The membranes used in reverse osmosis (RO) cannot be used indefinitely. Leaks in the membrane do occur and the product water flow rate and conductivity must be monitored on a continual basis. Only 25-50% of the volume of feed water is turned into product water. The rest of the feed water becomes a waste product. This has environmental and economic effects. The membrane of the RO unit must remain wet throughout its period of use, generally 1-2 years. The unit cannot be left with the flow stopped, as this will result in the growth of bacteria, the hydrolysis of the membrane, and the production of pyrogens. When out of operation, the RO unit must be kept filled with a sterilant.

DEIONIZATION

Deionization (DI) is the process by which ionized minerals and salts are removed from a solution. Feed water must be cleared of ionized minerals and salts. During deionization, the resin beads in the filter exchange positively charged ions for hydrogen ions. Hydroxide ions are formed by the exchange of negatively charged ions. The resulting hydrogen ions and hydroxide ions combine, and water is produced. Water with high ionic purity is created by deionization. The process does not, however, remove bacteria or pyrogens. Deionizers may encourage the growth of bacteria and endotoxins, as these may grow in the resin bed. Submicron filtration or ultrafiltration should be used with deionization to remove any existing bacteria and endotoxins. Deionization is accomplished with a DI unit.

TREATING WATER WITH ULTRAVIOLET LIGHT

Ultraviolet light is a type of radiation. It is used to purify water for use in dialysis. Ultraviolet light kills microorganisms by penetrating their cell wall and altering their DNA (deoxyribonucleic acid). The UV light source used in treating water for dialysis is covered in a protective quartz sleeve. The water is directed through a flow chamber and exposed to the UV radiation. The water must be reasonably calm, and clear and without suspended particles. Ultraviolet light does not penetrate murky liquid. Suspended particles in a liquid can supply a hiding place for microorganisms where

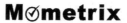

the ultraviolet light cannot reach. It is important to note that ultraviolet light cannot destroy endotoxins.

Maintain, Monitor, and Evaluate Systems

MONITORING THE EFFECTIVENESS OF WATER TREATMENT SYSTEMS

Tests used to check the effectiveness of water treatment include the following:

- **Bacterial culturing** is conducted to determine if bacteria are present in the product water. The colony count in the product water is measured at 24 and 48 hours. A bacterial culture is also used to test the dialysate.
- The **conductivity** of the feed and product water is tested to determine the ion content. Ion content is measured with a pHoenix meter or a handheld meter. The pHoenix digital dialysis meter also measures the pH of the water and the temperature.
- The water is tested for **resistivity**. Resistivity measures the efficiency of ion removal by a deionizer. High resistivity equals low conductivity.
- The water is tested for **hardness**.
- **TDS (total dissolved solids)** is a measurement of the total number of ions in a solution. It can be determined with a handheld meter. This test checks the efficiency of the RO membranes. TDS is expressed in terms of parts per million.

OBTAINING CULTURES OF WATER AND HEMODIALYSIS EFFLUENT

Cultures of the water supply and dialysate are carried out to determine if the effluent is contaminated with pathogenic organisms, such as bacteria. According to CMS guidelines, samples should be taken prior to disinfection ("worst case"). Water that should be tested include that used to reprocess chemicals, rinse water, stored water, water after it leaves the RO unit, at different points in the distribution loop (beginning, middle, end), water used for making concentrate solutions, and water used to make dialysate at the point of entry and (for effluent) at exit. The **culture procedure steps** include:

- Cleanse the outside of the sample port with alcohol solution and let completely dry.
- Run water for 60 seconds before collecting a sample in a sterile container.
- Using a pipette, transfer 0.1-0.5 mL of fluid from the sterile container onto a culture medium, using the membrane filter technique or direct application.
- Process samples within 2 hours or store for up to 24 hours in a refrigerator and then process.

TESTING METHODOLOGY FOR CULTURING SAMPLES

AAMI/ANSI guidelines recommend culturing a 0.3-1.0 mL sample for 168 hours at 17-23 °C using a low-nutrient agar medium. Incubation time has been extended and temperature decreased to allow for more bacteria to be identified. Culture methods include membrane filtration, spread plate assays, or pour plate assays. Millipore devices are acceptable only if duplicate samples are sent to an outside lab annually for comparison. Endotoxin testing should be performed by the LAL method. If any test results meet or exceed the action level, then the technician must isolate the problem, notify the nurse and physician, and take corrective action. The technician and Quality Assurance manager must evaluate trends from previous results. Trends must be continuously monitored, as slowly climbing levels can be early indicators of a problem with the water system.

COMMON CHEMICAL CONTAMINANTS THAT MAY CAUSE COMPLICATIONS

There are many contaminants other than bacteria and endotoxins in water that can cause complications during dialysis. The hemodialysis tech must conduct tests for chemical contaminants in water at the beginning of each shift. Three **common chemical contaminants** are:

Chemical	AAMI Standard Allowable Amount	Signs & Symptoms of Contamination
Chloramines (chlorine and ammonia byproduct)	0.1 mg/L chloramines; total chlorine not to exceed 0.5 mg/L. Formula for calculating chloramines levels is: Total chlorine – free chlorine = chloramines	Hemolysis, chest pain, abnormal heart rhythm, nausea, and vomiting
Nitrates (from fertilizers)	2 mg/L	
Copper (from copper pipe leachate)	0.1 mg/L	

MONITORING THE WATER TREATMENT TEMPERATURE-BLENDING VALVE

The temperature-blending valve mixes hot and cold water to achieve a specific water temperature, usually in conjunction with a water heater. This piece of equipment should be fitted with a thermometer. Raising the temperature of the water to around 77 °F allows reverse osmosis machines to operate most efficiently. Most of the time when the temperature blending valves fail, more hot water will be delivered than cold, and the water temperature will begin to rise. The technician must monitor output temperature and record it on a daily basis.

MONITORING THE DEPTH FILTRATION DEVICES

Depth filters use multiple layers of media in different sizes to remove particles from the water. Each layer of media is able to trap different sizes of particles, from large specks of dirt to microscopic bacteria. The pressure of these devices should be monitored pre-filter and post-filter. A pressure drop of more than 10 psi across the filter may mean that the media is clogged with sediment and should be backflushed or replaced. If a backflush timer is present, it should be set to go into operation during the facility's off hours.

MONITORING THE ACID FEED PUMP

In areas where the pH of the feed water is high (alkaline), the technician must introduce acid into the water to bring the level into a pH range of 7.0-8.0. The pH is monitored with a testing meter or strip held in a sampling port downstream from the acid pump. The acid feed system should be placed before the multi-media filters to prevent aluminum precipitation. Both audible and visual alarms should be in place to warn of unsafe changes in pH. Independent tests of pH are required on a daily basis.

MONITORING THE DEIONIZATION SYSTEM

Water pressure is monitored before and after each DI tank that is in use. Changes of more than 10 psi from the baseline measurements can indicate that the tanks are becoming filled with particles. If a holding tank is used with a DI system, the flow in the distribution system should be no less than 3 feet per second. The DI system should also be monitored for bacterial and chemical contamination to meet AAMI standards, just as with an RO system. It is vitally important that all staff who monitor water quality understand what the different LED lights mean on DI systems.

Monitoring the Drain System

There should be a minimum of a 1-inch gap between the machine's drain lines and the building's drain pipes. This gap prevents sewage from being taken up by the machine's drain lines, should the sewage system back up. The gap also prevents direct contact of the drain line with the drain pipe. The drain lines sometimes attract fruit flies, which can be an infection control problem in dialysis units. Pouring bleach or a commercially prepared gel-type product into the drain lines on a regular basis can help diminish the fruit fly population.

Medicare Conditions of Participation for Chlorine Testing

The Medicare Conditions of Participation state that testing for chloramines/chlorine should be conducted by a water treatment technician on every shift. If there are no set shifts, then testing must be conducted at intervals of no greater than 4 hours. The acceptable limit for chlorine is 0.5 mg/L and the level of chloramines should be 0.1 mg/L. It is important that the technician has the water system up and running for 15-20 minutes before performing the chlorine test. The water should be tested at the point where it leaves the first carbon tank. If any chlorine is present, then a sample should be taken at the point immediately after water leaves the second tank. If chlorine is present at this point, then dialysis should be stopped at the facility due to the risk of hemolytic anemia to the patients from blood exposure to chlorine.

Monitoring Product Water

Product water is the water that is produced after it has completed the water treatment process. This water must meet AAMI standards for chemical composition. The standards state that monitoring is required once per year, but the medical director is responsible to see that water quality is maintained at all times. In order to stay in compliance with AAMI standards, test product water quarterly. Obtain samples immediately after the RO or DI system. Product water should be monitored continuously for conductivity in RO water or resistivity in DI water.

Monitoring Feed Water

Feed water is untreated water that enters the dialysis unit. Feed water should be analyzed by a lab at least four times a year so that its chemical composition is known, and to account for seasonal variations. Monitor the back-up water plan as well. Failure to monitor the back-up water on a quarterly basis is a frequent cause of citations by certifying agencies. The feed water sample should be taken from its source, before it enters any part of the treatment system. Monitoring the feed water assures that the water system is able to clear the water of contaminants.

Monitoring the Water Softener System

Four elements to be monitored in the water softening system include:

- The AAMI standard for post-softener hardness is 1 grain per gallon or 17.24 ppm.
- Pressure should be monitored pre and post softener. After a baseline for the device is established, if the pressure drops by more than 10 psi, then the unit should be backflushed.
- Water softeners exchange sodium ions for calcium and magnesium. Therefore, an adequate amount of salt in the brine tank is essential for operation. Also, check for the development of a salt bridge, a formation of salt crystals across the tank that causes it to appear full when it is actually empty underneath.
- The regeneration timer should be set to go into operation during the unit's off hours. Verify that the unit is not set to regenerate during a dialysis session.

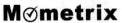

WATER SUPPLY TESTING AFTER AN ADVERSE EVENT

An **adverse event (AE)** is an unintended, unfavorable occurrence caused by medical intervention (iatrogenesis) that threatens the patient's life, or requires in-patent hospitalization, or extends the patient's length of stay, or causes a birth defect or lasting disability. When an adverse event occurs, the technician draws blood cultures, dialysate cultures, and dialysate endotoxin levels from the patient. The rationale for this is that blood and dialysate cultures will give a positive result if bacteria are present, but will be negative if endotoxins are present. Endotoxin testing that is performed in the dialysis unit gives results in about an hour, as opposed to a wait of up to 72 hours for final bacterial cultures from blood and dialysate. Assay cultures that cannot be completed within 1-2 hours may be refrigerated for 24 hours. Cultures held longer than 24 hours are inaccurate.

DOCUMENTING WATER TREATMENT SYSTEM QUALITY CHECKS

Water quality is a vitally important safety and Quality Assurance issue. Meticulously document water treatment system checks, because the surveyors will ask to see them during their accreditation visit. The unit must have well-documented checks to keep its operating license. The surveyors consider performing checks but failing to document them is the same as not doing them. Documentation is the only proof that the water program is running safely and efficiently. Keep a log book of all checks performed. The person performing the checks must sign or initial beside the date and time. Do not leave blanks in the log book. If the entry does not apply, write 'N/A' next to it, or strike a single line through the space. The error must still be readable, the error corrected, and initialed.

Infection Control

Maintain a Clean and Safe Patient Environment

SIGNIFICANT BLOOD BORNE PATHOGENS IN DIALYSIS

A pathogen is a microbe that is capable of producing disease. Bloodborne pathogens that can be transmitted in a dialysis unit include:

Type	Example
Viruses	HIV/AIDS; Hepatitis B, C, and D; cytomegalovirus (CMV); and herpes
Parasites	Malaria, Chagas disease, African sleeping sickness, and toxoplasmosis
Bacteria	Sepsis from *Staphylococcus, Streptococcus,* or *Yersinia enterocolitica;* brucellosis; cutaneous gonorrhea; diphtheria; tuberculosis; mycoplasma caviae; Rocky Mountain spotted fever
Prions	Variant Creutzfeldt-Jakob disease (vCJD, or mad cow disease)
Spirochetes	Syphilis, yaws, and Lyme disease

Hepatitis B is much more infectious than HIV due to the higher concentration of hepatitis virus in the blood. There is a 30% chance the technician will develop Hepatitis B following a needle stick injury, a 10% chance of Hepatitis C, and a 0.3% chance of HIV infection. All dialysis personnel are entitled to free vaccination against Hepatitis B, and should encourage their patients to receive the vaccine as well. Current statistics reflect that only 20% of dialysis patients receive vaccination for Hepatitis B.

INFECTION CONTROL PROCEDURES

HIV VS. HEPATITIS VIRULENCE

Virulence refers to the severity of the disease that a pathogen produces. HIV is much less of a threat in the dialysis setting than Hepatitis B. However, many Hepatitis B positive patients are also co-infected with HIV, syphilis, and tuberculosis (TB). HIV dies after about 10 minutes of contact with the air. HIV is very easily destroyed by a one-minute exposure to sodium hypochlorite (bleach) solution. By contrast, Hepatitis B lives 7 days on inanimate surfaces. The HIV **viral load** (concentration) ranges from 10-10,000 viruses per milliliter of blood. Hepatitis B contains 100 million viruses per milliliter of blood. The CDC suggests preparing a 1:10 dilution of household bleach daily as an inexpensive, effective way to kill HIV and HBV on surfaces. The CDC warns that aluminum equipment is corroded by bleach, and milder disinfectants (e.g., glutaraldehyde) may be more appropriate for sensitive equipment.

PRECAUTIONS FOR HIV

Standard (universal) precautions are all that is necessary when caring for patients with HIV in the dialysis unit. The rationale is that the AIDS virus:

- Is not transmitted on environmental surfaces.
- Has a lower viral load in the blood than Hepatitis B.
- Is not transmitted by airborne routes or mosquitoes.

The position of the CDC on reuse of dialyzers is that it may be performed if the technician uses the proper technique; however, many units decide not to reuse dialyzers on HIV patients. If a dialysis room surface comes into contact with a known infectious virus, such as HIV or Hepatitis B, wash the area thoroughly with a 1:10 dilution of bleach and water and immediately inform the supervisor.

POST-HIV EXPOSURE FOR HEALTHCARE WORKERS

If a healthcare worker is exposed to HIV, he or she should notify their supervisor. The Centers for Disease Control and Prevention (CDC) recommends counseling and medical assessment after exposure. HIV-antibody tests should be conducted immediately and at regular intervals for a period of at least six months. Precautions should be taken by the healthcare worker to prevent secondary infection. Provisional recommendations have been issued regarding post-exposure prophylaxis. A three-drug post-exposure prophylaxis is recommended (upon healthcare worker discretion and request) using antiviral therapy, but should be discontinued if testing proves that the exposed healthcare worker is HIV-negative.

HEPATITIS B

Hepatitis B, also called HBV, is easily transmitted by infected individuals because of the concentration of the virus carried in the blood. The virus can also survive at room temperature, outside the body, for many days. This means the virus can survive on environmental surfaces. The virus can be transmitted directly from penetration of the skin by sharp contaminated objects, or by exposure of broken skin or mucous membranes to contaminated blood. It can also be transmitted indirectly from contaminated surfaces in the environment. It is strongly recommended that healthcare workers be vaccinated against the virus. The series of vaccinations recommended is 85-97% effective in preventing infection after exposure. If protective levels of antibodies have formed after vaccination, booster shots are not necessary for healthy individuals. Dialysis patients, however, may need booster shots after antibody levels have decreased.

SYMPTOMS

Hepatitis B causes both acute and chronic infection. HBV can be transmitted by sexual contact, an infected birth mother to the fetus, sharing needles or grooming equipment, touching infected wounds, sharing food pre-chewed by an infected person, and contaminated blood transfusions. Patients who display immediate symptoms of infection after HBV exposure are considered to have **fulminant hepatitis**, which is life-threatening. Generally though, HBV takes 45-160 days to incubate. During its incubation time, the patient may not show any symptoms. Infants, children, and immunosuppressed patients may not show any signs of infection at all. Symptomatic patients may present with anorexia (loss of appetite), malaise (a generalized unwell feeling), nausea and vomiting, abdominal pain, jaundice (yellowed skin and sclera of the eyes), skin rashes, and joint pain. 90% of patients have normal immune systems that eventually conquer HBV and they will be immune to further attacks. 10% of patients have immune deficiencies and will go on to become chronically infected with the Hepatitis B virus for 6 months to a lifetime, and are infectious **carriers** even when they are asymptomatic.

LONG-TERM CONSEQUENCES OF CHRONIC HEPATITIS B INFECTION

Many patients who have **chronic Hepatitis B infection** are asymptomatic (have no symptoms at all); however:

- 66% of chronic HBV patients will develop chronic liver disease.
- 15-20% of patients will die prematurely from cirrhosis or liver cancer.
- They are carriers who are likely to transmit HBV on to other persons.

There were about 21,000 new cases of acute HBV infection in the US in 2018. According to the CDC approximately 862,000 Americans have chronic Hepatitis B. The complications of HBV are a very high price to pay for a disease that is largely preventable by a routine vaccination program. Hepatitis B vaccine has been part of the recommended vaccination schedule of infants and young children since 1991, and that led to an 80% decline in HBV infection. Nevertheless, some parents still neglect children's vaccinations, or do not permit them for religious reasons. The majority of dialysis patients are elderly and live on a fixed income, so often they have not been vaccinated.

PRECAUTIONS WHEN DIALYZING PATIENTS WITH HEPATITIS B

Patients who are HBsAg positive should be dialyzed in a separate room, away from the main treatment area, and on dedicated equipment that is only used on HBsAg positive patients. Do not place these patients on the reuse program. Preferably, staff should not care for HBsAg positive patients and unvaccinated patients, or patients with no documented antibodies to the virus, during the same shift. Staff can care for Hepatitis B positive patients and patients with known antibodies during the same shift. Flag the patient's chart to warn other staff members. To prevent spreading the infection:

- Wash hands frequently.
- Do not remove anything from the isolation area.
- Wear gowns, gloves, and face protection.
- Remove PPE and wash before leaving the isolation area.
- Incinerate contaminated laundry.
- Decontaminate unsoiled laundry before washing.
- Never eat, drink, or smoke in a dialysis area.

CONTROLLING THE SPREAD OF HEPATITIS B

Because the Hepatitis B virus is able to remain alive on environmental surfaces for at least 7 days in the dialysis unit setting, it has been recovered from doorknobs, clamps, machine controls and scissors. Any surface that is not routinely cleaned can become a reservoir for Hepatitis B virus and can allow the staff to transmit the virus to other patients through contact with these surfaces. In fact, most Hepatitis B outbreaks in dialysis units have been traced to contact with contaminated environmental surfaces and supplies, by the use of single dose medication vials by more than one patient, or by preparing medications in the centralized treatment area. Staff members who care for both Hepatitis B positive patients and those that are susceptible at the same time are disease vectors for their patients. The head nurse will try to reschedule staff and patients to avoid this situation.

RISK FACTORS FOR ACQUIRING HEPATITIS B IN DIALYSIS CENTERS

According to the CDC, the risk factors for patients acquiring the Hepatitis B virus include:

- A dialysis facility that has at least one patient with Hepatitis B who is not under isolation (blood precautions).
- Less than 50% of the patient population has been vaccinated against the Hepatitis B virus.

The CDC recommends routine screening for Hepatitis B virus be conducted for all patients on admission to the dialysis unit, and then periodically thereafter. Vaccination programs for patients and staff should be instituted and monitored by Occupational Health. All staff working with dialysis patients should encourage them to be vaccinated against the Hepatitis B virus, and impress upon them the importance of completing the vaccine series of two or three injections.

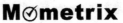

PREVENTING THE SPREAD OF HEPATITIS B VIA EQUIPMENT AND SUPPLIES

The Centers for Disease Control (CDC) recommends that the dialysis unit provides known Hepatitis B patients with supplies and equipment that are dedicated for their use only. This includes clamps, blood pressure cuffs and stethoscopes. Dedicated items should not leave the designated Hepatitis B stations. In addition, the CDC recommends that one individual supply tray be dedicated to each patient, regardless of the patient's hepatitis status. The technician must disinfect equipment between patients, using an appropriate antimicrobial disinfectant. Housekeeping must send an environmental aide to clean the dialysis area on a regular basis. Dialysis staff must don gloves before touching a patient or any hemodialysis equipment. Dialysis staff must doff the used gloves, wash hands or use an alcohol sanitizer, and don a new pair before going to another patient station. These simple precautionary measures have been shown to reduce the transmission of Hepatitis B by 70-80%.

HEPATITIS C

Hepatitis C virus was formerly called non-A non-B. It causes hemolytic anemia and the bleeding disease idiopathic thrombocytopenic purpura (ITP or Werlhof's disease). A Hepatitis C patient is unlikely to be approved for a kidney transplant because he/she will probably develop cirrhosis of the liver. After a needlestick injury containing infected blood, a technician has a 10% chance of contracting Hepatitis C. Hepatitis C is the most common type of hepatitis contracted following blood transfusion. Vaccination is available to prevent Hepatitis A and B, but there is no vaccine to prevent Hepatitis C. Hepatitis C is less virulent than Hepatitis B. The viral load for Hepatitis C is approximately 1,000 viruses per milliliter of blood. The virus lives for at least 16 hours and up to 4 days outside of its host. Both staff and patients in dialysis units are at increased risk for acquiring Hepatitis C. Use standard precautions to prevent spreading the virus. Hepatitis C patients with controlled liver enzymes need not be restricted from reuse programs.

GUIDELINES FOR MONITORING HEPATITIS C

All Hepatitis C patients should have the liver enzyme tests ALT and AST performed monthly. Normal ALT is 5-35 IU/L. Normal AST is 5-40 IU/L. Liver enzymes are a sensitive indicator for hepatitis of any type, and are correlated with Hepatitis C antibodies. Hepatitis C antibodies indicate that a person has been exposed to the Hepatitis C virus, but cannot detect whether the infection is past or current. If the patient does not have elevated liver enzymes, then obtain anti-HCV levels at 6-month intervals. If the patient has negative anti-HCV levels and elevated liver enzymes, repeat the anti-HCV level. If elevated liver enzymes are sustained and the patient still tests anti-HCV negative, then obtain an HCV RNA level. HCV RNA is a direct test for the Hepatitis C virus.

TUBERCULOSIS

Individuals with tuberculosis contact the bacteria *Mycobacterium tuberculosis* from airborne particles or *Mycobacterium bovis* from infected milk. Elderly people exposed to TB in their youth can develop active TB infection decades afterward.

- **Latent TB**: No signs or symptoms occur. Healthy immune response prevents further bacterial spread 2-10 weeks following exposure. These individuals will test positive Mantoux skin test or QFT-G blood test. 10% of exposed persons with positive Mantoux tests develop active TB infection. Offer prophylaxis with isoniazid (INH) and rifapentine.

- **Active TB**: Lungs appear "moth-eaten" on x-ray; 15% of patients develop infection in the GI tract, genitals, bones, meninges, or lymph nodes. Signs and symptoms include a persistent cough lasting longer than three weeks sometimes accompanied by blood-tinged sputum, exhaustion, fever, weight loss, and night sweats. Sputum test for TB confirms Mantoux or QFT-G. Active TB patients are infectious and transmit *Mycobacterium tuberculosis* bacteria through respiratory secretions.

SCREENING

All individuals working for a dialysis facility should be screened for tuberculosis when hired. Screening for TB is carried out at least once a year but often more frequently. Frequency of screening is determined by the risk. Institutions with a high-risk patient population will screen more frequently for the disease. New patients should be screened before their first dialysis treatment. If the patient was tested within the last year, this may not be necessary unless risk factors are present. The 2-step Mantoux test is recommended by the Centers for Disease Control and Prevention (CDC) for baseline screening. In the 2-step Mantoux test, 0.1 mL of purified protein derivative (PPD) is injected intradermally and then the injection site is assessed for induration after 48-72 hours. The test is repeated in 1-3 weeks. If a case of TB is noted in the patient population, or among the facility personnel, the testing schedule should be altered as needed.

TRANSMISSION

Pulmonary tuberculosis (TB) is spread by **airborne particles** infected with *Mycobacterium tuberculosis*. TB was called consumption in 1900, when 80% of US population contracted it by age 20, and it caused most deaths. In the 1940's, streptomycin brought TB under control. In the 1980's, TB increased with the decline of the public health system, crowded prisons and homeless shelters, lack of immigrant screening, and AIDS. If a patient is suspected to have TB, place a surgical mask over the patient's face to prevent the spread of contaminated particles. Wear a HEPA mask (N95, SCBA or PAPR) for self- protection, and ventilate the treatment room. Adjust air conditioning and heaters so they do not recirculate air. TB is most prevalent among people living in crowded conditions; the elderly; those of African-American, Hispanic, Asian, and Pacific Islander decent; and people with AIDS, alcoholism, and IV drug abuse.

IMPLICATIONS OF TB FOR DIALYSIS UNITS

In 2019, the Centers for Disease Control and Prevention (CDC) reported approximately 8,900 cases of TB in the US (2020 numbers may be skewed due to the onset of COVID-19). This marks a decline from 2000, when more than 16,000 cases of TB were reported. The CDC reported 92 cases of multi-drug resistant tuberculosis (MDR TB) in 2019. Treatment of MDR TB is dependent upon the drugs to which the case is resistant, making it very complicated. Tuberculosis outbreaks occur in facilities where close human-to-human contact occurs, such as prisons, dialysis units, and hospitals. Patients with active TB should not be dialyzed in out-patient dialysis centers. Patients with active infections should be dialyzed in a hospital isolation unit with negative airflow capability. Regulations for ESRD freestanding dialysis units state the unit must be able to access backup hospital facilities. After the TB patient receives treatment and is no longer considered infectious, then out-patient dialysis in the clinic setting may resume.

MRSA

MRSA (methicillin-resistant *staphylococcus aureus*) is a drug-resistant organism found in healthcare facilities in the United States. MRSA has become resistant, through mutation, to the commonly used antibiotics. Individuals with suppressed immune systems are vulnerable to MRSA infection. MRSA is usually transmitted by the hands of healthcare workers. The disease is transferred to the healthcare worker's hands after he or she touches an infected patient or a patient who carries the organism. The organism can then be transferred to another patient. Individuals can become infected through openings in the skin, such as wounds and pressure sores. Some individuals are carriers and harbor the organism in the nasal passages or on the skin. MRSA may also survive on environmental surfaces and contaminate these surfaces.

DIALYZING PATIENTS WITH MRSA AND VRE

The transmission of MRSA can be controlled by use of standard precautions. The prevention of the spread of VRE may take extra precautions. If a patient with VRE has undressed wounds that are draining, diarrhea, incontinence, or poor hygiene, he or she should be dialyzed in a separate room. A dedicated set of noncritical equipment should be used for patients with VRE or patients who are carriers of VRE. This equipment may be used for only a single patient or for a group of patients infected with, or carrying, the organism. If equipment used on patients with VRE is to be used for other patients, it must be cleaned and disinfected first.

NEEDLESTICK INJURIES

Hepatitis C is the bloodborne disease most likely to be transmitted to a healthcare worker by needlestick. It is uncommon to be exposed to HIV through a needlestick. Healthcare facilities have a protocol in place that must be followed in the event of a needlestick. Prophylactic treatment should be considered if a healthcare worker suffers a significant needlestick. A significant needlestick involves the production of a bleeding wound. Healthcare employers must follow certain safety regulations. The sharp devices used at the workplace must be engineered for safety. A log of contaminated needlesticks must be maintained by the employer. The details of the injury must be recorded. Staff must be trained in the safe use of all sharp devices.

PATHOGENS RESPONSIBLE FOR CENTRAL VENOUS ACCESS INFECTIONS

Central venous access infections are the most common type of infection in dialysis patients, and account for one-third of all infections. Fistulas and Gore-Tex grafts are far less likely to develop bacterial contamination, so the nephrologist will be eager for the surgeon to replace the central venous access with a safer access. If the central access site is infected, it will produce pain, heat, and drainage. Infection can spread to the bloodstream, causing sepsis and death from shock. The most common pathogens associated with catheter-related infections, in descending order, are:

- Staphylococcus aureus
- Coagulase-negative staphylococci (CNS)
- Gram-negative bacilli
- Nonstaphylococcal Gram-positive cocci (including enterococci)
- Fungal infections

HANDWASHING

Pathogens are commonly transferred between individuals in a healthcare facility by the hands. The risk of spreading contaminants can be significantly reduced by handwashing. The caregiver should wash his or her hands upon entering the patient care area, when leaving the patient care area, before and after gloving, and after touching a surface in the environment without gloves. All caregivers should follow the handwashing guidelines established by the Centers for Disease Control and Prevention (CDC). Alcohol-based rubs can be used instead of soap and water unless the hands are visibly dirty or contaminated. Traditional handwashing with soap and water should involve a 15-second wash followed by a rinse. When using an alcohol-based rub, the caregiver should apply the rub to the palm of the hand. The hands should then be rubbed together until the product is absorbed and the hands dry.

USING ALCOHOL-BASED SANITIZERS

Alcohol rubs are less irritating to the hands than repeated washing. If alcohol-based rubs are used correctly, and are of adequate concentration, they kill twice as much bacteria in the same amount of time as hand washing. The safety officer is required to train and observe the hemodialysis technician for compliance. Here is the correct procedure for hand disinfection:

1. Rub hands briskly for at least 15 seconds with an alcohol-based rub, such as Purell®, before and after contact with a patient or after removal of gloves.
2. All hand surfaces should be thoroughly coated with the alcohol rub, including between the fingers, the wrists, and under the nails, and then the hands rubbed together until the solution evaporates.
3. Do not rinse the hands.

NOTE: Alcohol-based rubs disinfect but do not mechanically clean hands, so hands that are dirty or contaminated with bodily fluids should be washed first with soap and water. Certain bacteria are resistant to alcohol-based rubs and require handwashing with soap and water, such as *Clostridioides difficile*.

CDC GUIDELINES FOR INFECTION CONTROL

PREVENTING CONTAMINATION OF MEDICAL AREAS

CDC's recommendations to prevent contamination of medical areas are as follows:

- Never prepare medications in the dialysis treatment area. They could be contaminated by backsplashes or aerosols. Prepare medications in a designated area, preferably a room with a closed door.
- No unrelated activities should take place in the medication room.
- Do not place biohazard containers, blood samples or other specimens, or contaminated supplies or equipment in the medication room.
- Do not wear the same gloves at a patient station and then in clean areas.
- Prepare medications in the medication room and take them to each patient individually.
- If using trays to deliver medications, they must be cleaned after each patient.
- Common medication carts should not be used in the treatment area.
- Medication vials that are marked for single use should only be punctured one time with a needle.

USE OF SUPPLIES AT DIALYSIS STATIONS

CDC's recommendations regarding the use of supplies at dialysis stations are as follows:

- Do not take common supply carts to individual dialysis stations. Any item that is taken to a patient station could potentially be contaminated with pathogens. This includes items that are placed atop the dialysis machine or in baskets on the side of the machine.
- All items that remain unused at the end of the patient's treatment must be one of the following:
  - Cleaned and disinfected by the technician
  - Designated for use on only one patient
  - Thrown away in the appropriate garbage container
- The technician must dispose of unopened packages of alcohol swabs, gauze, or syringes when dialysis ends.

- The technician must doff gloves and wash hands before removing supplies from the clean utility area. Hand washing is imperative because gloves can allow contamination of the hands through undetected holes in the glove or by fluid rolling beneath the cuff. Hands must be clean when obtaining items from a clean area, due to the potential for touching and contaminating other items while selecting needed supplies.

Using Dialysis Precautions and Implementing Isolation Procedures

STANDARD PRECAUTIONS

It is recommended that standard precautions be taken to help prevent the transmission of bloodborne diseases to healthcare workers. Bloodborne diseases include human immunodeficiency virus (HIV) and hepatitis B virus (HBV). It may not be possible to identify patients with a bloodborne disease. Standard precautions state that it should be assumed that all patients are potentially infectious. Blood, body fluids containing blood, semen, and vaginal secretions may carry bloodborne diseases. Standard precautions involve the use of personal protective equipment (PPE) to prevent contact with pathogens. PPE is also called barrier precautions. Gloves, masks, protective eyewear, and impervious gowns are types of PPE.

FACE PROTECTION

Face protection is accomplished with a mask and goggles or a face shield. Eye glasses are not sufficient protection. For maximal eye protection, wear goggles with wrap-around shields that protect the eyes from the sides. Use face protection any time the eyes could be splashed or aerosolized body fluids could be inhaled. Wear face protection when doing the following:

- Centrifuging specimens.
- Beginning the dialysis procedure.
- Performing venipuncture.
- Troubleshooting the patient access.
- Discontinuing dialysis.

If blood does contact the eyes or mucous membranes, flush them immediately with copious amounts of lukewarm, running water. Inform the supervisor and fill out the incident report form within 24 hours of the accident. If the patient has a bloodborne infection like Hepatitis B or AIDS, then the hemodialysis technician is entitled to free prophylactic drugs, regular follow-up, and counseling from Occupational Health.

GLOVES

Gloves are worn for touching blood and body fluids, mucous membranes, and broken skin of all patients. They are also used for handling items contaminated with blood or body fluids, and for any vascular access procedure. Gloves are changed and the hands washed after contact with each patient. Clean gloves are applied before the next patient contact. Gloves are also changed immediately after visible soiling or handling of infectious waste containers. Hands should be washed before touching patient charts or environmental surfaces, such as machine controls or equipment. Never handle a patient chart with gloves on. If the hemodialysis technician or the patient is allergic to latex, wear non-latex gloves.

DISPOSAL OF BIOHAZARD WASTE AND SHARPS

Patient and dialysis **safety precautions** include:

- **Hazardous wastes** (including dialyzers): Spill kits must be available on the unit and PPE must be worn when handling hazardous wastes and chemicals, such as germicides. The hemodialysis technician must be trained in the proper use, storage, and disposal of chemicals in use. Hazardous waste disposal should be in double bags and labeled/color-coded as hazardous.
- **Sharps**: Sealed leak- and puncture-proof sharps containers should be available at each dialysis station or treatment area. Recapping should be avoided and used needles disposed of immediately. The sharps container should be removed and disposed of when three-quarters full.

ISOLATION PRECAUTIONS AND DISINFECTION OF ISOLATION EQUIPMENT

Isolation precautions vary according to the type of infection:

- **Hepatitis B**: Provide treatment wearing PPE in dedicated isolation room with dedicated equipment (including instruments and supplies), and new dialyzer. Staff caring for patients with HBV should not also care for patients who are susceptible (HBSag/HBSAB negative).
- **Hepatitis C and HIV**: Utilize standard hemodialysis safety procedures.
- **MRSA, VRE, and *C. Diff*:** Place patients as far away from other patients as possible, use standard precautions, and always wear a gown over clothing and change gown before and after caring for the infected patient. Use dedicated equipment, such as BP cuff and stethoscope.
- **Tuberculosis**: Carry out dialysis in isolation negative-pressure room and wear N95 disposable respirator while providing care. The patient must wear a face mask when outside of the isolation room.
- **COVID-19**: Patients should be provided dialysis in an isolation negative pressure room. The CDC recommends that dialysis staff try to provide treatment and monitor the patient from outside of the patient room, through a window, if possible. This minimizes exposure time to the patient. Dialysis staff should wear an N95 mask, gown, gloves, and a face shield or goggles while providing care and the patient, if able to tolerate a mask, should also wear a mask when the dialysis staff is present.

Disposable equipment should be disposed of as hazardous waste and all non-disposable equipment cleaned and disinfected or sterilized according to manufacturer's guidelines. All surfaces and equipment in patient area or room must be cleaned and disinfected.

Education and Professional Development

Educate the Patient

NUTRITION

Diet may be used as therapy for individuals with renal disease. The dietitian works with the nephrologist and makes recommendations regarding the patient's diet. The dietitian monitors the patient and makes adjustments to the diet as necessary. Diet may delay the need to put the patient on dialysis by slowing the progress of renal disease. Diet can prevent or reduce many of the complications that can occur as a result of renal disease. For example, restricting the patient's intake of phosphorus can help prevent the development of bone disease. The incidence of morbidity and mortality can be decreased by an adequate intake of protein and calories. Diet can be modified to reflect the individual needs of patients with renal disease.

DIET PRIOR TO INITIATION OF DIALYSIS

The patient's diet is assessed before dialysis treatment begins and adjustments are made. There are several goals of diet therapy. It is hoped that an appropriate diet will delay the need for dialysis by slowing the progression of renal disease. Limitations on the intake of protein, and an adequate intake of calories, can help decrease the level of nitrogenous wastes produced and can also help manage symptoms of uremia. The patient should be encouraged to maintain a high enough caloric intake so that that protein contained within the body is not catabolized. Phosphorus can be controlled to an extent by limiting the intake of phosphorus in foods. Before dialysis is initiated, hypertension can be managed by limiting the intake of sodium. It is not usually necessary to limit potassium intake until dialysis treatments have started.

SODIUM INTAKE

Sodium intake must be **strictly monitored** in patients with renal disease. For most hemodialysis patients, a dietary sodium intake of 2300 mg per day (100 mmol/day) is acceptable. The patient's blood pressure, output of urine, and level of fluid retention should be monitored as these can be adversely affected by sodium levels. Fluid retention is evidenced by the development of edema. The dietary intake can be adjusted as necessary. Patients in ESRD usually develop hypertension as a result of increased fluid volume. If the patient is hypertensive, his or her dry weight should be monitored on a continuing basis. Occasionally patients with renal disease develop renin-mediated hypertension. For these patients, hypertensive medications are necessary.

POTASSIUM INTAKE

Potassium is found in most foods. Some fruits and vegetables are very high in potassium. Dietary limitations of potassium should be based on the patient with goals to maintain serum potassium levels within normal range. Often, the dietary intake of potassium may be limited after urine output has dropped to less than 1 L per day. In some cases, dietary intake of potassium should be restricted before the output of urine falls to this extent. Most patients with kidney disease can safely ingest 2730 mg of potassium, which equals 70 mEq. The height and weight of the patient, along with the amount of potassium in the dialysis fluid, affect the amount of potassium that can be safely ingested as part of the diet. Hyperkalemia may be caused by factors other than diet. Severe acidosis, constipation, catabolism, an insufficiency of insulin, and certain medications may contribute to the development of hyperkalemia.

CALORIC INTAKE AND FAT INTAKE

Dyslipidemia is commonly seen in patients with renal disease. In these patients, dyslipidemia usually presents as hypertriglyceridemia in conjunction with low high-density lipoprotein cholesterol and normal total serum cholesterol. Some patients with renal disease, however, may have elevated serum cholesterol, which means serum cholesterol higher than 200 mg/dL. This group of individuals may benefit from a diet low in cholesterol and fat. Hypertriglyceridemia may be worsened by obesity. In patients who are obese, weight control may help keep triglyceride levels under control. Aerobic exercise on a continuing basis may help keep cholesterol and triglyceride levels under control. Triglyceride levels may also be lowered by including carnitine and fish oil supplements in the diet. Is has been suggested that patients with renal disease may be at higher risk for developing atherosclerosis. Dialysis has a moderate effect in improving dyslipidemia.

PROTEIN INTAKE

It has been recommended that the **protein intake of hemodialysis patients should be in the range of 1.0-1.2 g/kg/day**. Patients who are lacking in protein should be at the upper end of the range. It is also recommended that 50% of the protein requirement be obtained from sources such as meat, fish, and poultry. This type of protein source contains proteins comprised of all the essential amino acids. These are called high biologic-value protein sources. Low biologic-value sources include fruits, vegetables, and grains. If the diet is carefully designed, adequate protein can be obtained from nonanimal sources. Patients with renal disease have higher protein requirements than individuals in the general population. This is due, in part, to the loss of amino acids during hemodialysis.

TREATMENT OPTIONS FOR THOSE UNABLE TO EAT

A patient with end-stage renal disease may be unable or unwilling to eat for several reasons. These reasons include the following: uremia caused by underdialysis, gastroparesis, depression, comorbid illness, gastrointestinal disturbances (i.e., constipation, nausea, vomiting), and side effects of medication. Each patient should be assessed and treated individually. Nutrient intake can be augmented by nutritional supplements. There are ways to increase food intake. For example, patients may be able to increase their food intake if they eat 5 small meals per day instead of 3 large meals. Medications to increase appetite may be useful. If the patient is unable to eat and his or her health is deteriorating, enteral nutrition may be considered. Intradialytic parenteral nutrition may be considered for those who continue to deteriorate.

PATIENT EDUCATION REGARDING PHYSICIAN'S ORDERS AND PRESCRIPTIONS

Patients must have a clear understanding regarding the physician's orders:

- **Personal hygiene**: Because of the risk of infection, patients must understand the importance of bathing regularly, wearing clean clothes, and washing hands frequently, especially if they are involved in self-care, such as inserting their own needles.
- **Self-care**: All aspects of care should be explained in detail to patients, and they should be encouraged to participate in self-care as much as possible to promote feelings of independence. Those who practice self-care are more likely to opt for in-home dialysis, which can allow for more frequent treatments and better control.
- **Treatment modalities**: Patients should understand different options for hemodialysis (graft, fistula, catheter), site (in-center, in-home) and frequency (daily, 3 days a week, 5 days a week).
- **Dialysis prescription**: Patients should understand the basis of the dialysis prescription, which will include the settings (flow rates, UF rates), the target ("dry") weight, and target Kt/V as well as the frequency and duration of treatments.

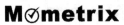

IMPACT OF DIALYSIS PRESCRIPTION ON NEUROPATHY

The dialysis prescription is the manner in which the treatment is administered. This varies according to the needs of the patient. Depending on the patient's response, the dialysis prescription may be adjusted as needed. The length of the treatment, type of dialyzer, dialysate, and rate of ultrafiltration constitute the dialysis prescription. Although the cause of neuropathy is unknown, it is suspected to result from the accumulation of medium- to large-size toxic molecules in the body that can be affected by many aspects of the dialysis prescription. These toxic molecules have not yet been identified. Neuropathy is rare if the dialysis prescription is adequate for the specific patient. If neuropathy is worsening, it suggests that the dialysis procedure needs to be intensified.

DISCHARGE INSTRUCTIONS

DIET

Discharge instructions for the hemodialysis patients regarding diet are critically important. Patients often develop malnutrition, which increases the risks of mortality, and the diet must be individualized. Patients must learn to read food labels. Patients generally require 1.2 g/kg per day (8-10 ounces per day) of protein because of protein loss during hemodialysis. However, this results in nitrogenous wastes that must be removed during treatment. Calorie intake must be sufficient to avoid loss of "real" weight (as opposed to fluid weight). Intake of electrolytes is limited, so patients must be aware of foods that should be avoided:

Electrolyte	Ideal Range	Foods With High Levels
Sodium	Usually ≤2000 mg/day	High sodium foods include salt, bottled sauces, salted snacks, ham, bacon, cured meats and luncheon meats, processed cheese, and most frozen, canned, and fast food.
Potassium	Maintain blood level at 3.5-5.0 mEq/L	High potassium foods include bananas, oranges, avocados, salt substitute, fresh cooked spinach, potatoes, sweet potatoes, nuts, beans, chocolate, dried fruits, and cantaloupe.
Calcium	<1000 mg/day	High calcium foods include dairy products, beans, lentils, dark leafy greens, fortified breakfast cereal, almonds, and seeds.
Phosphorus	800-1000 mg/day	Foods that are high in phosphorus are those also high in protein, such as meat, fish, poultry, beans, nuts, and dairy products.

FLUID INTAKE AND MEDICATIONS

As part of **discharge instructions**, patients should be educated about:

- **Fluid intake**: Allowable intake may vary depending on whether the person is still producing urine. Those who produce little or no urine have more fluid restriction because fluid retention is greater, and it's more difficult to reach dry weight. Patients should be taught to measure fluids, estimate fluids in foods, weigh daily, and to estimate their fluid gain based on the weight and the physical effects of retained fluids (edema, shortness of breath, cramps) and should learn to pay attention to their bodies. Generally, most patients are instructed to avoid gaining more than 1 kg/day (2.2 pounds).

- **Medications**: Patients must understand the names of all medications, the dosages, the frequency, and the purpose as well as possible adverse effects. Medications commonly taken by those on dialysis include erythropoietin (to increase production of red blood cells), iron (to produce red blood cells), vitamin D (to help control levels of calcium, phosphorus, and parathyroid hormone), and phosphorus binders (to help decrease levels of phosphorus). Patients may also take antihistamines to relieve itching, vitamin B complex, and folic acid.

REHABILITATION ACTIVITIES

The role the hemodialysis technician has related to participation in patient rehabilitation activities, such as exercise regimens, includes:

- Question patients about the types of daily activities they engage in (cooking, cleaning, driving, watering the yard, working) that may promote fitness.
- Question patients about their routine practice or participation in exercise programs.
- Encourage patients to exercise on a regular basis and to participate in exercise programs available to patients.
- Suggest simple at-home exercises patients can do as part of routine activities.
- Educate patients about the benefits of exercise in maintaining physical functioning, preventing complications, and promoting a feeling of well-being.
- Encourage and allow patients to do as much as possible for themselves.
- Assist patients to walk with their walkers rather than utilizing a wheelchair to save time.
- Encourage patients to do simple stretching exercises, such as of the legs, while they are undergoing dialysis.

CONSTIPATION

Patients with end-stage renal disease often become constipated and/or develop fecal impactions because of a number of factors including diet, fluid restriction, and the regular ingestion of phosphate binders. Older patients on dialysis tend to develop diverticula of the colon. Patients on dialysis have a high rate of diverticulitis and perforation of the bowel. Incorrect use of enemas may cause hematomas and perforation of the bowel. Individuals with end-stage renal disease and constipation should use cathartics and laxatives carefully. Many laxatives contain magnesium, phosphorus, and/or potassium, and should be avoided by individuals with end-stage renal disease. Stool softeners make voiding the bowels easier, and the use of these is permissible.

FEMALE FERTILITY

Infertility is common among women on dialysis. The pregnancy rate for women on dialysis is low. The reason for this is unclear, but the problem is probably due to an endocrine abnormality. Although the fetal survival rate in pregnant women on dialysis is below normal, it has improved. Up to 80% of these pregnancies are successful and produce a live infant, but risk of preterm labor and neonates with low birth weight, in addition to other complications in both the fetus and mother, are higher. Increasing the frequency of dialysis treatments leads to longer gestation and increases the chances that the fetus will be delivered successfully. Intense hemodialysis aids in controlling maternal intravascular volume and decreases the risk that the mother will develop hypotension resulting from excessive ultrafiltration. Men on dialysis can also have fertility problems, usually due to poor sperm formation.

IMPACT OF CHRONIC DIALYSIS ON MENSTRUAL CYCLE

Uremic syndrome in women often results in the **cessation of the menstrual cycle.** Although cases of pregnancy in women on dialysis have been reported, research suggests that the majority of women of child-bearing age on dialysis do not ovulate. The majority of women of child-bearing age who are on dialysis suffer from amenorrhea or oligomenorrhea that is anovulatory in nature. Many women suffer from galactorrhea. These abnormalities of the menstrual cycle may be due to disruptions in the hormonal feedback mechanisms. Excessive menstrual flow should be reported, as this problem can lead to undesirable blood loss. Women of child-bearing age on peritoneal dialysis will exhibit blood-tinged dialysate during menstruation and ovulation

SEXUAL DYSFUNCTION

Sexual dysfunction is a common occurrence in individuals on maintenance dialysis. In men on maintenance dialysis, uremia leads to a drop in libido and impotence. Research suggests that as many as 60% of men on maintenance dialysis suffer from total or partial impotence. Research studies suggest that impotence associated with maintenance dialysis may have an unknown organic basis 50-70% of the time. Medication may be a contributing factor to the incidence of impotence in men on maintenance dialysis. Decreased libido and reduced ability to reach orgasm are also seen in women with chronic kidney disease. Hemodialysis may exacerbate sexual difficulties in individuals with chronic kidney disease.

PSYCHOLOGICAL IMPACT OF DIALYSIS
STAGES OF ADJUSTMENT TO DIALYSIS

There are three stages of adjustment associated with the need for dialysis: the honeymoon period, the period of disenchantment and discouragement, and the period of long-term adaptation. These stages are not always linear. Different patients spend different amounts of time in a particular stage, and patients may shift back and forth between the stages.

- The **honeymoon period** occurs at the start of dialysis and last weeks or months. The patient feels better physically and mentally and views dialysis positively.
- The **period of disenchantment and discouragement** is characterized by loss of hope and confidence. This stage may last 3-12 months. It occurs when the patient is faced with the reality of his or her limitations.
- The **period of long-term adaptation** is the last stage. The patient has come to terms with his or her limitations and the realities of dialysis. The patient may alternate between contentment and depression.

PSYCHOLOGICAL CONSEQUENCES OF DIALYSIS

Patients differ in their reactions to dialysis. Some patients suffer a gradual health decline and become depressed. These patients are at increased risk for suicide. Some maintain good health on dialysis and do not experience depression. No predictive factors related to patient response to dialysis have been found. A patient's past history of coping provides the best indication of his or her response to dialysis. The dialysis patient's personality traits can be evaluated to help predict his or her response to treatment. The mental health professional on the patient's dialysis team will conduct an in-depth analysis of the patient and the patient's family. The outcome of the evaluation can be used to develop a treatment plan, which may include psychosocial counseling.

STRESS

End-stage renal disease places patients and their families under severe stress. Individuals with end-stage renal disease may experience lack of control over their lives, sexual dysfunction, guilt, depression, and loss of self-esteem. Job loss may lead to a sense of worthlessness. Finances may suffer due to the illness. Family relationships change as responsibilities shift. Patients may deny their limitations or refuse to adhere to treatment. This can reduce the patient's quality of life and increase the risk of complications and death. It is important that noncompliance with the dialysis regimen be recognized promptly. The dialysis team must be ready to refer the patient to an appropriate resource person, such as a psychiatrist or social worker.

EMOTIONAL PROBLEMS IN FAMILY MEMBERS OF PATIENTS ON DIALYSIS

The family members of patients on dialysis often experience **anxiety**. This is particularly true at the start of dialysis. The stresses of having a family member on dialysis may cause other reactions. The family members may feel **resentment** toward the patient due to the financial drain and demands placed on them. A patient on dialysis may become **demanding, aggressive, and antagonistic** toward his or her family members. In response, the family members may become hostile toward the patient. The family members may then feel **guilty** for having negative feelings. Staff of the dialysis facility can help the situation by the use of active listening techniques. Staff members can reassure the family members that their feelings are normal and understandable.

NONADHERENCE

There are a number of ways that a patient may exhibit non-adherence to the dialysis regimen. Patients may refuse to adhere to the prescribed diet. This can adversely affect the patient's health and increase the risk of death. Patients may ingest fluids in excess of recommended amounts. This could adversely affect health by increasing fluid load. Patients may not adequately care for their vascular or peritoneal access. This could cause a clot in the line or an infection of the access. A patient may skip treatments or shorten the time of a treatment. The patient is then not receiving adequate dialysis. Non-adherent behavior can result in a number of problems including malnutrition, nerve cell damage or death, and cardiac failure. Non-adherent behavior may be viewed as passive suicide, as it can result in death.

PATIENT EDUCATION ON CHRONIC KIDNEY DISEASE

Chronic kidney disease (CKD) is defined by the National Kidney Foundation (NKF) as damage to the kidney lasting for 3 months or longer, or by a decreased level of kidney function for a period of 3 months or longer. Decreased level of kidney function is defined as a glomerular filtration rate (GFR) of less than 60 mL/min/1.73 m^2. Kidney damage is characterized by pathologic irregularities or markers that indicate damage. Markers indicating damage may be found by blood or urine tests, or by imaging studies. Chronic kidney disease is diagnosed according to whether or not physical damage is present and according to the level of kidney function present. The type of kidney disease does not affect the determination of chronic kidney disease.

COURSE

The course of chronic kidney disease varies considerably between patients. It can take months or years to reach end-stage renal disease. The number of nephrons still functioning decreases as the course of the disease progresses. The still-functioning nephrons must take on more and more solute load as the disease progresses. Azotemia and uremia eventually occur when the level of solute that can be cleared has been reached. The body is able to adapt to a certain extent to the chemical abnormalities. End-stage renal disease is diagnosed when the kidney function permanently decreases to the point that the kidneys can no longer remove waste products and maintain the body's normal fluid and chemical balances. End-stage kidney disease can develop slowly or rapidly.

STAGES

The stages of chronic kidney disease are determined according to the level at which the kidneys are functioning. The stages of chronic kidney disease are defined by cut-off levels of continuous measures of kidney function. Therefore, the stages are somewhat arbitrary. This definition of stages, however, provides clinical guidelines for treatment.

Determining the presence and stage of chronic kidney disease not does mean that a diagnosis has been made. The cause and extent of the disease must be determined. In addition, the extent of any kidney damage and the level of function must be assessed. The patient must be assessed for any possible complications associated with the kidney disease, and any comorbid conditions.

Glomerular filtration rate (GFR) is accepted to be the best method of measuring kidney function. Chronic kidney disease (CKD) is divided into 5 stages based on severity of the condition. CKD is staged according to the level of the GFR.

- Stage 1 CKD involves kidney damage with normal or increased filtration. GFR is greater than 90.
- Stage 2 CKD involves a mild decrease in function with a GFR of 60-89.
- Stage 3 CKD is divided into two sub-stages:
  - Stage 3a CKD: A mild to moderate decrease in function with a GFR of 45-59.
  - Stage 3b CKD: A moderate to severe decrease in function with a GFR of 30-44.
- Stage 4 CKD involves severe loss of kidney function with a GFR of 15-29.
- Stage 5 CKD is kidney failure and involves a GFR of less than 15. Dialysis is required at this stage. Stage 5 kidney disease is also called end-stage renal disease (ESRD).

RISK FACTORS

CKD is becoming more prevalent in the United States and is an increasing cause of death. The National Kidney Foundation has determined a number of risk factors for the development of CKD. Risk factors include age, family history, diabetes, hypertension, and population of origin. Older individuals tend to have more health problems than younger people, leaving them more susceptible to kidney damage. In addition, kidney function decreases with age. Some kidney diseases are strongly hereditary, and certain heritable conditions create a susceptibility to kidney disease. Individuals with poorly controlled diabetes are at higher risk for developing kidney disease. Hypertension can both cause CKD and occur as a result of CKD. Hypertension can cause or exacerbate kidney disease by damaging blood vessels. African Americans, Native Americans, Latinos, and Pacific Islanders are more likely to develop the disease than individuals from other populations.

STEPS TO MANAGE CKD

The National Kidney Foundation recommends **screening for all individuals** to determine if they are at risk for developing chronic kidney disease (CKD), and further screening for those who are at risk. Risk factors identified by the National Kidney Foundation include hypertension, diabetes, age of 60 or older, and family history of kidney failure requiring dialysis/transplant. The **goal** of clinical treatment of CKD is to slow the progression of the disease and to ease symptoms.

- In patients with Stage 1 CKD, treatment is planned after diagnosis. Any comorbid conditions are treated. Management is aimed at slowing the progression of the disease and preventing cardiovascular problems.
- In patients with Stage 2 CKD, the progression of the disease is monitored.
- In patients with Stage 3 CKD, complications may arise. The complications are evaluated and treated.
- In patients with Stage 4 CKD, the patient is prepared for kidney replacement therapy.
- In patients with Stage 5 CKD, treatment involves a kidney transplant if uremia is present.

END-STAGE RENAL DISEASE

End-stage renal disease (ESRD) involves the complete, or almost complete, loss of kidney function. The kidneys lose their ability to excrete wastes, concentrate urine, and regulate the level of electrolytes. Chronic kidney disease (CKD) may be managed for a period of time by diet, the use of medications, restricting the intake of sodium, and controlling phosphates. CKD is progressive and as kidney function worsens over time, the conditions can no longer be managed. When the kidneys lose all but 10-15% of their normal function, dialysis or transplantation is necessary for the patient's survival. Without treatment, the accumulation of fluids and waste products in the body will cause the patient's death.

PATIENT EDUCATION REGARDING END-STAGE RENAL DISEASE

Patient education regarding end-stage renal disease includes:

- **Complications**: Anemia may occur because of inadequate production of red blood cells. If the kidneys are unable to effectively remove phosphorus, hyperphosphatemia may leach calcium from the bones and the body may be unable to effectively utilize vitamin D, resulting in osteoporosis. Heart disease may result from increased blood pressure and coronary artery disease (from excess homocysteine and high levels of calcium and phosphorus). Fluid retention may result in generalized edema, respiratory distress, and tachycardia.
- **Treatment**: Generally, includes either hemodialysis or peritoneal dialysis or kidney transplant and dietary restrictions. Some patients may opt for medical management to provide supportive care.
- **Dietary restrictions**: Patients generally need to restrict intake of fluids, sodium, potassium, and phosphorus. Patients should avoid food that are pickled or high in salt/sodium (soy, sauces, prepared foods, processed meats, canned vegetables) and should not add salt to foods. Patients may also be advised to limit protein (pre-dialysis) and simple carbohydrates (sugar, flour), especially patients with diabetes.

INCIDENCE OF INFECTIONS IN ESRD

Infection is a common cause of death in individuals with end-stage renal disease. Some patients with end-stage renal disease have leukocyte abnormalities. These abnormalities include a low white blood cell count. Granulocytes do not respond normally to the presence of infection. Individuals with end-stage renal disease are particularly susceptible to developing infections due to several factors. Many patients with end-stage renal disease suffer from malnutrition. They may have immune system deficits. Invasive measures necessary for the treatment of end-stage renal disease often leave patients with conditions making them susceptible to infection. The use of intravenous iron in patients with end-stage renal disease is also associated with the development of infection. Infection may be difficult to diagnose in individuals with end-stage renal disease because hypothermia is not uncommon in these patients. Furthermore, an infection in a patient with end-stage renal disease may not cause a fever because urea decreases body temperature.

RESPIRATORY PROBLEMS IN ESRD

Individuals with renal disease experience a number of types of associated respiratory difficulties.

- Patients with acute kidney injury have a higher incidence of **pulmonary edema**. The pulmonary edema results from fluid accumulation and left ventricular dysfunction.
- **Tuberculosis** affecting the lungs occurs approximately 10 times more often in patients on hemodialysis than in the general population.

- Patients with renal disease may develop **metabolic acidosis**, which can cause Kussmaul respirations. Kussmaul respirations occur as the body tries to rid itself of excess carbon dioxide. Kussmaul respirations are characterized by abnormally deep and fast breaths. Metabolic acidosis is a condition in which excess hydrogen ions accumulate in the blood. The diseased kidneys are unable to clear these ions from the body.

GLUCOSE METABOLISM IN ESRD

Whether or not they have diabetes, glucose metabolism is abnormal in individuals with end-stage renal disease. The cellular sensitivity to insulin is decreased from normal levels in individuals with end-stage renal disease. Although serum glucose is almost at normal levels after a glucose load, the speed of decline is slower than normal. The peripheral cellular resistance to insulin is particularly severe in individuals who developed end-stage renal disease as a result of type-1 diabetes. In this case, large and frequent swings between hypoglycemia and hyperglycemia often occur. Dialysis improves the situation somewhat, but wide variations in blood glucose levels still occur. Appropriate insulin levels may be difficult to establish in this population because of the kidneys' inability to efficiently metabolize insulin. Diabetic end-stage renal disease usually involves type 2 diabetes. Obesity is often a contributing factor, and the situation can be improved with weight reduction. Oral hypoglycemic agents may help.

PROTEIN METABOLISM IN ESRD

Patients with end-stage renal disease often have **protein calorie malnutrition**, which results in the reduction of lean tissue mass. The condition develops because of poor protein intake. Insufficient protein and calories are taken in to maintain the body. Low serum albumin also results from poor protein intake. The patient with this disorder may appear emaciated, but the condition may be masked by edema. In this condition, the levels of a number of nonessential amino acids are elevated and levels of some essential polypeptides are reduced. Symptoms of protein calorie malnutrition include weight loss, bradycardia, hypothermia, and low basal metabolism. Protein calorie malnutrition is also called kwashiorkor. Although the condition is a prominent characteristic of end-stage renal disease, it also has other known causes.

LIPID METABOLISM IN ESRD

Individuals with end-stage renal disease often have **type 4 hyperlipoproteinemia.** Type 4 hyperlipoproteinemia is also called **hypertriglyceridemia**. The terms hyperlipoproteinemia and hyperlipidemia are interchangeable. Type 4 hyperlipoproteinemia is a lipid disorder. This condition is characterized by increased blood levels of very low-density lipoproteins (VLDL). Triglycerides make up VLDLs. Type 4 hyperlipoproteinemia involves elevated triglycerides only. The condition is common and is also associated with obesity and diabetes. Unlike other types of hyperlipoproteinemia, type 4 hyperlipoproteinemia does not appear to place the affected individual at higher risk for heart disease, but the risk of pancreatitis is increased. The pancreas manufactures insulin and substances required for digestion.

HEMATOCRIT AND HEMOGLOBIN IN ESRD

Hemoglobin and hematocrit are used to test for anemia. If hematocrit and hemoglobin are low, epoetin alfa may be prescribed. Patients with end-stage renal disease generally have **low hematocrit and hemoglobin** because erythropoietin production is low. A low hematocrit level can result from a reduction in red blood cell production, dialysis-related blood loss, and/or a reduced lifespan of red blood cells. In patients with renal disease, a normal hematocrit value is 30-36%. Signs and symptoms associated with a low hematocrit value include heart palpitations, fatigue, dyspnea, and chest pain. Hemoglobin contains the iron that is needed to transport oxygen throughout the body's tissues. A desirable hemoglobin value in patients with end-stage renal disease is 11-12 g/dL.

IMPACT OF RENAL FAILURE ON BODY SYSTEMS
IMPACT OF RENAL FAILURE ON INTEGUMENTARY SYSTEM

The integumentary system includes the skin, nails, hair, the tissue directly underneath the skin, and various glands. Patients with end-stage renal disease often have brittle hair and nails and dry skin. These changes in the integumentary system occur because the activity of the sweat and sebaceous glands decrease in individuals with end-stage renal disease. Individuals with end-stage renal disease may develop calcium deposits in the skin. This causes intractable pruritus. The patient with this condition may damage his or her skin severely trying to relieve the itching. Uremic frost is a condition seen in patients with advanced, untreated uremia. In this condition, the deposition of urea crystal precipitates causes the skin to look frosty. Increased deposition of carotenes, along with skin pallor from anemia, may cause the skin to take on a tan-yellow color. Ecchymosis, a skin discoloration caused by the escape of blood into the tissues, is common.

ELEVATED BUN IN DIALYSIS PATIENTS

Increased blood urea nitrogen (BUN) can be caused by renal insufficiency, ingesting large amounts of protein in the diet, digesting blood released in the gastrointestinal tract, dehydration, infection, trauma, or fever. Increased blood nitrogen urea in a dialysis patient can indicate that the dialysis prescription requires adjustment. It may be necessary to increase the time spent on the dialyzer, to increase the rate of blood flow during dialysis, or to use a larger dialyzer. Symptoms of elevated levels of blood urea nitrogen include fatigue, sleeplessness, irritability, nausea, itchy skin, and a change in the senses of taste and smell. Patients with end-stage renal disease have a higher blood urea nitrogen level than individuals in the general population. While the normal level of blood urea nitrogen in the general population ranges from 7-18 mg/dL, the normal level in a patient with end-stage renal disease is 60-100 mg/dL.

UREMIA

Uremic syndrome, also called uremia, is a set of symptoms caused by disordered biochemical processes resulting from renal failure. Renal failure causes many toxic substances to be retained in the body. More than 200 toxins have been identified that contribute to uremic syndrome. Level of blood urea is positively correlated with the severity of uremic symptoms. As urea levels increase, symptoms worsen. The accumulation of urea in the blood contributes to uremic syndrome, but other toxins play a more important role in the development of the syndrome. A buildup of urea in the blood can cause lethargy, anorexia, and insomnia. Uremia includes a number of conditions including azotemia, acidosis, hyperkalemia, hypertension, anemia, and hypokalemia.

PERICARDITIS

Pericarditis is a cardiovascular disorder that occurs as a complication of end-stage renal disease. The pericardium is a fluid-filled, membranous, double-layer sac that surrounds the heart. The pericardial sac contains 15-20 mL of fluid. The fluid between the 2 membranes of the sac acts as a lubricant and permits the layers to slide over each other as the heart contracts. The uremic toxins, fluid accumulation, and infectious agents (bacteria and viruses) can irritate the pericardium, causing pain and fluid accumulation. Fluid accumulation around the heart is called pericardial effusion. The signs and symptoms of pericarditis include prolonged sharp chest pain, low-grade fever, fatigue, coughing, hiccups, and pericardial friction rub. Pericardial friction rub is caused when the layers of the pericardium rub together instead of sliding freely. The chest pain worsens with deep breaths, swallowing, and coughing. Pain eases when the patient sits and leans forward.

DIAGNOSIS AND TREATMENT

Although complications from pericarditis rarely occur, possible complications include pericardial effusion, pericardial tamponade, and constrictive pericarditis. Pericarditis is diagnosed by physical examination, electrocardiogram (ECG), x-ray, blood tests, and echocardiogram. Pericardial rub is heard during systole at the lower left sternal border on auscultation of the chest. An electrocardiogram may show elevated ST segments. The echocardiogram can be used to ascertain if pericardial effusion is developing. An x-ray of the chest can be used to check for fluid buildup. Pericarditis can have a number of causes. It is necessary to treat the underlying cause of the pericarditis. If caused by chronic kidney disease, pericarditis is treated by aggressive dialysis therapy with ultrafiltration. This is necessary to rid the body of uremic toxins and excess fluid. Steroidal and nonsteroidal anti-inflammatory drugs may be administered to decrease inflammation.

PERICARDIAL EFFUSION

Pericardial effusion is a complication of pericarditis. It can also be the result of kidney failure. It involves the buildup of abnormal amounts of fluid in the pericardial space. Pericardial effusion usually occurs due to an imbalance between the production and resorption of the fluid in the pericardial cavity. It can also occur when fluid enters the pericardial cavity through a structural abnormality. There is normally 15-50 mL of pericardial fluid in the pericardial cavity. The signs and symptoms of pericardial effusion include fluid retention, low blood pressure, chest pain, fever, hypotension, shortness of breath, and bloody pericardial fluid. Pericardial friction rub may not be present. The underlying cause of the condition must be treated.

PERICARDIAL TAMPONADE

Pericardial tamponade is an extreme case of pericardial effusion. The condition may have a slow or fast onset. There is limited space in the pericardial cavity. If enough fluid accumulates in the pericardial cavity, it places pressure on the heart. This pressure impairs heart function. Pericardial tamponade is a life-threatening condition. In the case of cardiac tamponade, the fluid must be drained from the pericardial space to relieve the pressure on the heart and restore normal function. To drain the fluid causing the pericardial tamponade, a needle is inserted through the chest wall into the pericardial space. It may be necessary to leave a drainage tube in place for a number of days. Surgical drainage may be required. The underlying cause of the pericardial tamponade must be treated.

ANEMIA

Individuals with uremia have a greater tendency to bleed than healthy individuals. This is due to a deficit in the production of platelets and a reduction in platelet quality. The hematologic defect most frequently seen among individuals with uremia, or individuals on dialysis, is anemia. Patients with uremia and patients on maintenance dialysis have significantly lower hematocrit values. The normal hematocrit for men is 46-52%. In women, the normal hematocrit ranges from 40-45%. Anemia in individuals with uremia and individuals on maintenance dialysis results from the reduced secretion of erythropoietin. The signs and symptoms of anemia in these populations include fatigue, pale skin, respiratory difficulties, and chest pain. Red blood cells have a much shorter lifespan in individuals with uremia.

CAUSES

Anemia has numerous causes, some more common than others. These causes include: low red blood cell production; a higher rate of red blood cell destruction; the inhibition of the actions of erythropoietin; chronic disease, including kidney disease; dialysis treatment; blood loss; iron deficiency; nutritionally inadequate diet; pregnancy; alcoholism; and abnormally high levels of

parathyroid hormone. Chronic kidney disease can interfere with the body's ability to produce sufficient numbers of red blood cells. Erythropoietin, a hormone produced by the kidneys, is responsible for stimulating the bone marrow to produce red blood cells. Patients with chronic kidney disease on dialysis may experience anemia. Dialysis treatment can result in the loss of blood, leading to anemia.

DIAGNOSIS AND TREATMENT

In their Dialysis Outcomes Quality Initiative (DOQI), the National Kidney Foundation makes recommendations for the **evaluation of patients on dialysis for anemia**. It is recommended that physicians conduct a detailed assessment of their male patients and postmenopausal female patients for anemia when the hemoglobin value drops below 37%. Women who have not reached menopause should be assessed for anemia when the HCT drops to lower than 33%. Evaluation for anemia in dialysis patients includes tests for iron deficiency and fecal blood loss. This ensures that the anemia is not due to some cause unrelated to the kidney disease. In a patient who has lost half of normal kidney function or more and has a low hemoglobin, then anemia is probably caused by a reduction in the production of erythropoietin.

Blood loss-induced anemia in the patient on dialysis can be minimized in a number of ways. Dialyzers should be pretested to ensure that they don't leak. The use and effects of heparin should be monitored to control clotting. Blood should be returned as completely as possible. Equipment should be properly maintained to prevent cell damage. The number of blood samples and the volume of blood taken should be kept to a minimum.

AZOTEMIA

Azotemia is an abnormal medical condition involving high levels of nitrogen-containing waste compounds in the blood. This is caused when the waste products produced by protein metabolism accumulate in the body. These waste compounds include such things as urea and creatinine. Azotemia is generally caused when the blood is not properly filtered by the kidneys. There are different of types of azotemia; azotemia is classified according to the cause of the condition. Prerenal azotemia is caused by an inadequate supply of blood to the kidneys. Postrenal azotemia is caused by the obstruction of urinary outflow. Some types of azotemia are caused by kidney disease. Trauma and disease of other organs of the body can also cause prerenal or postrenal azotemia.

HYPERTENSION

Hypertension, high blood pressure, is defined as blood pressure greater than 130/80 mmHg. Individuals with chronic kidney disease often exhibit hypertension. The hypertension can be the result of the kidney disease or be the cause of the kidney disease. Volume overload, an increased secretion of renin, uremic toxins, sodium in the diet, and secondary hyperparathyroidism can result in hypertension. There are 2 stages of high blood pressure. In stage 1, the systolic pressure ranges from 130-139 while the diastolic pressure ranges from 80-89. In stage 2, the systolic pressure is greater than 140 while the diastolic pressure is 90 or greater. In a patient with chronic kidney disease, hypertension is treated by medication and nonpharmacologic treatments. There are different categories of antihypertensive drugs and their mechanisms of action differ. More than one type of antihypertensive drug may be prescribed to treat the same patient.

EDUCATION FOR CHILDREN ON DIALYSIS
CAUSES OF CKD AND AKI IN CHILDREN

Causes of chronic kidney disease in children differ than those for chronic kidney disease in adults. Approximately two-thirds of the chronic kidney disease cases involving children result from congenital abnormalities of the urinary tract or hereditary diseases. About one-third of cases of

Copyright © Mometrix Media. You have been licensed one copy of this document for personal use only. Any other reproduction or redistribution is strictly prohibited. All rights reserved. This content is provided for test preparation purposes only and does not imply an endorsement by Mometrix of any particular political, scientific, or religious point of view.

chronic kidney disease in children result from acquired forms of glomerulonephropathy. The typical causes of kidney disease in adults rarely apply to children.

In children, acute kidney injury is typically caused by hypoperfusion of the kidney. Hypoperfusion of the kidney has a number of causes including septic shock, low blood pressure, severe dehydration, and significant acute blood loss. The hypotension causes acute tubular necrosis. Acute tubular necrosis can also occur in children and in adults due to the actions of nephrotoxic drugs.

EXTRACORPOREAL VOLUME IN A CHILD ON DIALYSIS

Generally, the extracorporeal volume in a child should not exceed 10% of the child's blood volume. After the treatment, the extracorporeal volume is returned to the body minus the amount needed for laboratory tests. If blood is needed for laboratory tests, the volume removed on a particular day should be limited to 3-5% of the child's total blood volume. When the extracorporeal blood must be kept under 12.5% of the blood volume, it is necessary to prime the system with a volume expander. Albuminized saline is often used for this purpose. When the extracorporeal blood is to exceed 12.5%, reconstituted blood may be used for priming. If the extracorporeal blood is to exceed 15%, then it is necessary to use reconstituted blood. Special products may be used to minimize the extracorporeal blood when dialyzing children. These lower the cost of dialysis by reducing the volume of reconstituted blood necessary.

TREATMENT OF CHILD WITH ESRD

Renal transplantation is the treatment of choice for children with end-stage renal disease. If chronic dialysis is necessary, home peritoneal dialysis is preferable to hemodialysis in a dialysis facility. Home peritoneal dialysis may not be possible for some patients. Existing techniques make hemodialysis in small children possible. The regimen needed for peritoneal dialysis, along with concerns about physical appearance, may cause some adolescents to choose hemodialysis over peritoneal dialysis.

The concentration of creatinine in the blood increases with increasing age and weight. Therefore, normal creatinine levels for adults and children differ. In children older than 2 years of age, creatinine concentration is normally in the range of 100-120 mL/min/1.73 m². End-stage renal disease is said to occur in children when creatinine concentration drops to less than 15 mL/min/1.73 m².

> **Review Video: <u>End-Stage Renal Disease</u>**
> Visit mometrix.com/academy and enter code: 869617

ACUTE KIDNEY INJURY
DEFINITION OF AKI

The term acute kidney injury (AKI) is used to describe a severe impairment of renal function with a sudden onset. The condition may occur over hours or days. A classical symptom of acute kidney injury is oliguria. Oliguria is defined as an output of less than 400 mL of urine in a 24-hour period. Anuria may also be a symptom. Anuria is the complete cessation of urine production. Nearly half of all cases of acute kidney injury do not involve oliguria. Nonoliguric kidney injury is easier to manage than oliguric kidney injury. The onset of nonoliguric acute kidney injury is not as quick, and the disease is not as severe as oliguric acute kidney injury.

DIAGNOSIS

Acute kidney injury is usually discovered in the intensive care units of hospitals. **Early signs** of acute kidney injury can be discovered by monitoring the patient's intake of fluid and the resulting urine output. Diagnosis is based on an **increase in serum creatinine** (by at least 0.3 mg/dL within 48 hours, or by at least 1.5 times the patient's baseline within the last 7 days) or a **decreased urine output** (0.5 mL/kg per hr for at least 6 hours). Testing the urine for electrolytes and the blood for solutes can also help in diagnosis. Serum urea can increase as much as 3.7-10.7 mmol/L per day. If the kidneys suffer extensive tissue damage, the blood levels of potassium, phosphate, sulfate, and hydrogen ions increase dramatically. If the acute kidney injury is the result of prerenal or postrenal causes, the condition can be reversed by correcting the underlying problem. Kidney function can often recover from intrinsic kidney injury, but the underlying cause that brought about the problem may not be correctable.

CAUSES

Acute kidney injury is divided into **three categories** based on cause. These are prerenal, intrarenal (intrinsic), and postrenal.

- **Prerenal acute kidney injury** involves a significantly reduced blood flow into the kidney. Kidney function is impaired by the reduced blood supply. The reduced blood flow can be caused by low extracellular fluid volume, heart failure, and blockage of the arteries serving the kidneys.
- **Intrinsic acute kidney injury** occurs when the kidney itself is damaged. Intrinsic acute kidney injury might occur with acute inflammation, compromised blood flow, or toxicity.
- **Postrenal acute kidney injury** involves an impeded flow of urine out of the kidneys. The ureter, bladder, or urethra can be blocked. Both prerenal and postrenal causes of acute kidney injury can often be corrected before the kidneys are damaged.

PHASES OF URINE OUTPUT

Patients with acute kidney injury may still excrete significant amounts of urine. This is called nonoliguric kidney injury. Patients with acute kidney injury generally go through several stages of urine output.

- **Oliguria** begins when the patient's urine output is less than 400 mL in a 24-hour period.
- **Anuria** is defined as a state in which the patient's urine output is less than 50 mL in a 24-hour period. Longer periods of oliguria/anuria indicate a poorer prognosis for recovery than patients with normal urine output.
- Recovery begins with the **diuretic phase**. The diuretic phase starts when the patient's urine output increases to 1 liter in a 24-hour period. Normal renal output returns gradually and output may reach 4-5 liters in a 24-hour period. The patient must be monitored at this stage to ensure that dehydration does not occur. Dehydration can cause hypoperfusion of the kidneys.

COMPLICATIONS

The complications of acute kidney injury include congestive heart failure and infection. Congestive heart failure occurs frequently in patients with acute kidney injury. High blood pressure, excess fluid volume, and anemia are common causes of congestive heart failure in acute kidney injury patients. In patients with acute kidney injury, the most common cause of mortality is infection. Uremia suppresses the immune system and increases the patient's risk of sepsis. Caregivers of a patient with acute kidney injury must adhere to aseptic technique at all times, especially at the start and finish of a dialysis session, during the insertion of an intravenous line, and during maintenance of the bladder catheter.

CLINICAL PRESENTATION

Acute kidney injury presents with signs and symptoms of **uremia**. These signs and symptoms include loss of appetite, nausea, vomiting, fatigue, lethargy, mental depression, sleepiness, headache, muscle cramps and twitches, sore gums, inflamed gums, abnormal skin sensations, discolored skin, and itchy skin.

The **biochemical changes** occurring in acute kidney injury include increased levels of urea and creatinine in the blood and a change in the electrolyte level. Acidosis and low blood pH may result from the increased concentration of hydrogen ions in the blood. Hyperkalemia, hypokalemia, hypocalcemia, hyperphosphatemia, and hypermagnesemia may occur during acute kidney injury.

SUPPORTING RENAL FUNCTION DURING AKI

Kidney function can be supported in a number of ways. Fluids may be lost during acute kidney injury and fluid replacement may be necessary. However, it may also be necessary to **restrict fluid intake** to prevent fluid buildup. A **specialized diet** may be prescribed that meets nutritional needs but does not strain the kidneys. **Medications** may be prescribed to relieve fluid buildup. Diuretics are no longer recommended as a measure to increase urine output, unless fluid overload is present. If the blockage in the kidney is causing the renal damage, a **catheter or stent** may be used to reroute the flow of urine.

DIALYSIS TO TREAT AKI

Acute kidney injury may be treated by hemodialysis, peritoneal dialysis, isolated ultrafiltration, continuous renal replacement therapy, and, in specific cases of drug-induced AKI, charcoal hemoperfusion. Patients with acute kidney injury may need dialysis every day, or every second day, until the kidneys heal and function is recovered. **Hemodialysis** is the most commonly used treatment for acute kidney injury and is recommended when fluid, electrolyte, and/or acid-base imbalances become life-threatening, but peritoneal dialysis is also an option. Although dialysis does not cure acute kidney injury or shorten its duration, it does help control blood pressure, correct fluid levels, and correct electrolyte imbalances. Dialysis requires the creation of an access site. The type of access depends on the type of dialysis. Approximately 50% of individuals who develop acute kidney injury recover kidney function. If kidney function is not regained, long-term dialysis or kidney transplantation are necessary.

INDICATIONS

Dialysis may be initiated when uremia, pulmonary edema, hyperkalemia, acidosis, neurological changes, drug overdose, and poisoning occur. Dialysis is started for patients with acute kidney injury when uremia becomes symptomatic regardless of blood urea nitrogen (BUN) and creatinine levels. Pulmonary edema can result from acute kidney injury and is life-threatening. Hyperkalemia in an acute kidney injury patient occurs as a result of the release of intracellular potassium. Dialysis can lower potassium levels. Acidosis is a metabolic disorder that occurs in acute kidney injury patients because the kidneys are unable to excrete hydrogen ions and reabsorb bicarbonate. Fluid overload becomes a problem. Neurological changes include headache, insomnia, sleepiness, mental confusion, seizures, and coma. Drug overdose and poisoning may require dialysis to remove the toxic molecules from the body.

FREQUENCY AND ACCESS USED

A **double-lumen venous catheter** is the type of access most often used with acute dialysis patients. The catheter may be inserted into the patient's right internal jugular vein, femoral vein, left internal jugular vein, or femoral vein (ordered according to KDIGO recommendations) using ultrasound guidance. If the catheter is placed in the subclavian or internal jugular vein, an x-ray must be taken to determine if the placement is correct. Incorrect placement could result in pneumothorax or hemothorax. If the patient requiring acute dialysis already has an arteriovenous fistula or graft, this access may be utilized. The access's patency must be determined first.

The patient's response to dialysis guides the frequency of the treatment. Hemodialysis may be carried out until the patient's blood levels of creatinine, urea nitrogen, and potassium are within acceptable limits. In addition, any acidosis must be resolved. It may be necessary to dialyze the patient daily for several days, particularly if volume overload is a problem.

PATIENT EDUCATION REGARDING ACUTE KIDNEY INJURY

Elements of patient education regarding treatment the patient should expect for acute kidney injury include:

- **Identifying and treating underlying cause**: This may involve multiple types of tests and different medications and treatments.
- **Maintaining fluid balance**: The patient will be carefully assessed (weight, central venous pressure, fluid intake/output) and may be on restricted fluids or receive diuretics or hypertonic sodium IV solutions for fluid overload.
- **Maintaining urinary output (prerenal causes of ARF)**: IV fluids and/or transfusions may be administered.
- **Monitoring for electrolyte imbalances**: Frequent blood draws for electrolyte levels and ECGs and/or cardiac monitoring for cardiac abnormalities will be conducted (especially related to hyperkalemia).
- **Dietary modifications**: High carbohydrate, low protein diets with restriction of foods high in potassium and phosphorus.
- **Hemodialysis** (usually temporary unless patient progresses to chronic renal failure): Catheter inserted for hemodialysis; frequency and duration varies according to severity of condition.

Engage in Professional Development

CONTINUING EDUCATION REQUIREMENTS FOR HEMODIALYSIS TECHNICIANS

The hemodialysis technician receives initial certification for a 4-year period and must recertify every 4 years thereafter. Recertification can be achieved by retaking the certification test, utilizing a one-time waiver of continuing education requirements, or completing 40 contact hours of **continuing education**:

- 30 of the contact hours must be from Group A providers (those that are BONENT approved): American Nephrology Nurses Association, Board of Nephrology Examiners Nursing and Technology, Nephrology Educators Network, Tukiendorf Training Institute, and the National Kidney Foundation.
- The remaining 10 contact ours can be from Group A or Group B and may include approved seminars, online courses, and home-study publications/short courses or workshops. Group B affiliated organizations include the American Heart Association, End State Renal Disease networks, American Kidney Foundation, and National Kidney Foundation. Approved journals include *Contemporary Dialysis & Nephrology, Dialysis & Transplantation, ANNA Journal, Nephrology News & Issues, Peritoneal Dialysis International, and National Association of Nephrology Technologists.*

MEDICATIONS IN DIALYSIS

DRUGS TO TREAT HYPERTENSION

There are different types of drugs used to treat hypertension. These include ACE inhibitors, angiotensin-receptor blockers (ARBs), beta-blockers, calcium channel blockers, and diuretics. The KDIGO 2021 guidelines recommend ACE inhibitors or ARBs as the first line pharmacological intervention for high blood pressure in CKD if lifestyle changes are ineffective. For individuals with a kidney transplant and high blood pressure, KDIGO recommends the use of and ARB or calcium channel blocker (CCB) as the first-line pharmacological intervention.

ACE inhibitors act to lower blood pressure by blocking an enzyme that causes blood vessels to contract. Blood pressure increases when blood vessels contract and lowers when blood vessels relax. ACE inhibitors also decrease the amount of salt contained in the body, which aids in decreasing blood pressure. ACE inhibitors have a protective effect on the kidneys and it is believed that they can stop renal disease from progressing. ACE inhibitors have a number of adverse effects. They can cause a persistent nonproductive cough, increased blood creatinine, rash, increased blood potassium, and angioedema.

> **Review Video: <u>Antihypertensives: ACE Inhibitors and ARBs</u>**
> Visit mometrix.com/academy and enter code: 525864

ARBs are sometimes given as an alternative to ACE inhibitors and are just as effective. ARBs lower blood pressure by blocking the effects of angiotensin II. Angiotensin II causes the blood vessels to constrict. The potential adverse effects of ARBs include headache, angioedema, and hyperkalemia.

Beta-blockers act to reduce blood pressure by reducing the speed at which nerve impulses travel through the heart. Decreasing the speed of nerve impulses through the heart reduces its need for blood and oxygen, and reduces its workload. This, in turn, decreases blood pressure. Possible side effects of beta-blockers include bradycardia (abnormally slow heartbeat), fatigue, weakness, dizziness, decreased saliva production, wheezing, cold extremities, and swelling in the extremities.

Calcium channel blockers (CCBs) lower blood pressure by slowing the passage of calcium into the heart and blood vessel walls. This action relaxes the blood vessels. Blood flows more easily through relaxed blood vessels, lowering blood pressure. The possible adverse reactions resulting from the intake of calcium channel blockers include headache, edema in the lower leg, fatigue, and gastrointestinal discomfort.

Diuretics are generally prescribed as one of the treatments for hypertension. Diuretics control high blood pressure by limiting water resorption, removing excess sodium from the body, and removing water from the body. The actions of diuretics cause a reduction in the total volume of water in the body and this reduces blood pressure. There are different types of diuretics and these exert their effects on different parts of the kidney. The side effects of diuretics include a reduction in the levels of some electrolytes, thirst, weakness, and frequent urination.

> **Review Video: <u>Calcium Channel Blockers and Antiarrhythmics</u>**
> Visit mometrix.com/academy and enter code: 942825
>
> **Review Video: <u>Diuretics</u>**
> Visit mometrix.com/academy and enter code: 373276

ANTICOAGULATION

Anticoagulation is the prevention or delay of blood clotting. Normally, clots develop when the blood comes in contact with a foreign surface or substance. Blood in the vascular system does not normally form clots, although this process may occur in some circumstances. Without intervention in the form of anticoagulants, blood would clot in the bloodlines and dialyzer unit.

Clotting occurs due to three factors: the damaged blood vessels pull back from the site of injury and contract; the blood platelets attach at the site of injury; or coagulation factors found in the blood interact to cause the formation of a blood clot. Blood does not clot in the vessels because of differences in the lining of the blood vessels and the surfaces of cells in the blood. The endothelium of the vessels is smooth, while the surfaces of the cells in the blood are gelatinous and contain large volumes of water.

> **Review Video: Antiplatelets and Thrombolytics**
> Visit mometrix.com/academy and enter code: 711284

HEPARIN

Heparin is an anticoagulant (blood thinner) with clinical uses. It is used in hemodialysis to prevent clots from forming in the bloodlines. Heparin can prevent the formation and growth of blood clots, but it cannot decrease the size of clots that already exist. Heparin is neutralized by strong alkalis, which take away its anticoagulant actions. Heparin binds with heparin cofactor, also called antithrombin III, forming heparin-antithrombin III. Heparin-antithrombin III prevents clotting by binding with and inactivating thrombin activated factor X and activated factor XI. Because of the presence of heparin, the conversion of prothrombin to thrombin and the conversion of fibrinogen to fibrin are prevented. Heparin has its greatest effects 5-10 minutes after its administration. When used in dialysis, the half-life of heparin is approximately 90 minutes.

> **Review Video: Heparin – An Injectable Anti-Coagulant**
> Visit mometrix.com/academy and enter code: 127426

TYPES OF HEPARIN AND DRUG INTERACTIONS WITH HEPARIN

Heparin is usually obtained from the intestinal mucosa of pigs or from the lungs of cattle. These types of heparin have slightly different properties. On a weight for weight basis, heparin obtained from pigs is a more potent anticoagulant than heparin derived from beef lungs. Because it is less expensive, the heparin most commonly used is that derived from the intestinal mucosa of pigs. Some patients may become allergic to porcine heparin. In these situations, it may be necessary to treat these patients with heparin derived from beef lung instead.

Some types of medications increase the anticoagulant properties of heparin and cause excessive bleeding. These medications include acetylsalicylic acid, non-steroidal anti-inflammatory drugs (NSAIDs), and dextran. Other drugs may decrease the effectiveness of heparin. These drugs include cardiac glycosides, tetracyclines, nicotine, and antihistamines. If nitroglycerin is administered intravenously to a patient on heparin, the partial thromboplastin time may decrease. When the nitroglycerin is discontinued, rebound results.

> **Review Video: NSAIDs and Their Adverse Side Effects**
> Visit mometrix.com/academy and enter code: 569064

Epoetin Alfa (EPO)

Epoetin alfa (EPO) is a recombinant form of erythropoietin placed on the market in 1989. It is commercially known as Epogen and Procrit. The product is used to treat patients with end-stage renal disease. EPO can increase hemoglobin to normal levels. EPO is administered when the patient's transferrin saturation (TSAT) is less than 30%. The goal of treatment with EPO is to raise the TSAT to greater than 30%. EPO is administered either intravenously or subcutaneously while the patient is at the dialysis facility immediately following a dialysis treatment. Patients may have a suboptimal response to EPO. The reason for this is usually iron deficiency. Other causes for a poor response to EPO include the following: infection and inflammation, chronic blood loss, osteitis fibrosa, aluminum toxicity, pathologies involving hemoglobin, a deficiency in folate or vitamin B12, multiple myeloma, malnutrition, and hemolysis.

Administration

EPO is administered intravenously or subcutaneously. The hemoglobin is measured before the start of dialysis to determine if anemia is present. The amount of EPO administered depends on the individual patient's TSAT, hemoglobin, and response to the substance. Sufficient amounts of iron and ferritin in the blood are necessary for EPO to have an effect. For use in dialysis patients, EPO is usually administered intravenously. It has been suggested by the Kidney Disease Outcomes Quality Initiative that the subcutaneous route of administration is just as effective or more effective as the intravenous route of administration. The Anemia Work Group prefers EPO to be administered subcutaneously. If EPO is used subcutaneously, the site of injection should be varied. Hemodialysis patients generally prefer EPO to be administered subcutaneously, as there are lower levels of discomfort involved.

Complications

EPO can cause **elevated blood pressure**. This occurs because the increased red blood cell mass causes the blood to become thicker than usual. This elevation in blood pressure usually occurs during the first 12 weeks of EPO therapy. At this time, the hemoglobin is still increasing. This complication is treatable with antihypertensive medications and dialysis, which removes fluids. The **effectiveness of hemodialysis decreases as the patient's hemoglobin increases**. This is due to the fact that the red blood cells tend to retain their toxins as they move through the dialyzer instead of releasing them. If the patient is receiving EPO, the caregiver and physician should monitor his or her blood chemistry. The dialysis prescription may require readjustment.

Blood Transfusions

Blood transfusions are not routinely administered to dialysis patients with a certain hemoglobin level. If the patient has lost a large volume of blood through a dialyzer leak or if the patient has a hemorrhage, the blood might need to be replaced. A blood transfusion will often relieve shortness of breath, fatigue, or angina. Because of possible complications that might arise from a transfusion, however, treating the anemia by increasing the dose of EPO is preferable to a transfusion. Some of the **possible complications** of blood transfusion are serious and include the following:

- Incompatibility reactions with the donor blood
- Allergic reactions to the donor blood
- Infections
- The development of preformed antibodies

Iron

Two measurements are used to determine if iron therapy is needed. The first measurement is called transferrin saturation (TSAT). To arrive at this measurement, the serum iron value is divided by the total iron binding capacity. This number is then multiplied by 100. TSAT is correlated with the amount of iron in the blood that can be used for erythropoiesis. KDIGO guidelines recommend considering supplemental iron if the TSAT is less than 30% and blood ferritin level is less than 500 ng/mL. A TSAT higher than 50% can be indicative of iron overload. The required iron is usually administered intravenously in patients on dialysis, and orally in patients with CKD that are not on dialysis. Iron overload, also called hematochromatosis, can occur as a result of repeated transfusions, excessive dietary iron, excessive iron replacement therapy, and genetic factors.

LEVOCARNITINE

Patients with end-stage renal disease who are receiving dialysis treatments may be lacking in an amino acid derivative called levocarnitine. Levocarnitine can be removed from the blood during dialysis. In addition, red meat and dairy products are a source of levocarnitine, and the diet of a dialysis patient may be deficient in these foods. Dialysis will result in a decrease in serum and skeletal muscle levocarnitine. This amino acid derivative is needed for the metabolism of fatty acids and for the production of energy. A number of organs in the body require levocarnitine for energy. These organs include the heart, liver, and kidneys. Supplements of levocarnitine are given to patients deficient in this amino acid derivative. Supplementation helps decrease muscle cramps and weakness. It also decreases hypotension that occurs during dialysis, increases cardiac output, and increases the capacity for exercise.

COMPLICATIONS SECONDARY TO MEDICATIONS

Antihypertensive medications can cause the patient to become hypotensive (faint from low blood pressure) during treatment. Examples of antihypertensives are: ACE inhibitors (Capoten, Lotensin, Vasotec), beta blockers (Inderal, Lopressor, Tenormin), and calcium channel blockers (Adalat, Cardizem, Norvasc).

Epogen (epoetin alpha) is an injectable drug to control anemia because patients with ESRD have kidneys that no longer produce erythropoietin needed to make red blood cells. Anemia causes extreme fatigue and requires blood transfusions. The doctor tries to keep the Epogen patient's hemoglobin in the 10-12 g/dL range to avoid blood clots that cause strokes, heart attacks, heart failure, or death. Tumors grow faster in patients taking Epogen. Patients taking Epogen need increased anticoagulants during dialysis. Epogen is associated with increased incidence of clotting in AV grafts, but not in native vessel fistulas. Epogen is also associated with hypertension (increased blood pressure), as the hematocrit rises and red blood cell mass increases.

IV iron during dialysis (also for anemia) can cause allergic reactions, hypotension, cramping, nausea, and headaches.

BODY MECHANICS FOR INJURY PREVENTION

The use of proper body mechanics is important to avoid common musculoskeletal injuries from repetitive actions, use of excessive force, and incorrect positioning/posture. Hemodialysis technicians should:

- Avoid bending over at the waist but rather squat, bending the hips and knees.
- Avoid turning when in the process of pushing, pulling, or lifting an item.
- Use appropriate transfer techniques, such as chair to chair transfers, slide boards, stretcher to chair or bed transfers and stand and pivot procedures.
- Use lift devices rather than manually lifting and ensure that the lift device is appropriate for the weight and size of the patient.
- Asking for help when needed to avoid unnecessary strain.

- Avoid reaching for prolonged periods of time, overhead, or more than 20 inches.
- Avoid pulling—push, roll, or slide instead.
- Avoid lifting—push, roll, or slide instead—and stand close to any object that must be lifted or carried.
- Maintain firm base of support with feet apart (shoulder width) to stabilize stance.

REDUCING FALL RISKS

The hemodialysis technician must take an active role in reducing risk of falls on the dialysis unit. Safety measures include:

- Encouraging and supporting a general culture of safety.
- Assessing and identifying patients who are particularly at risk of falls, such as those with diabetes, history of previous falls, motor impairment, or vision impairment.
- Recognizing that all dialysis patients have some risk of falls.
- Assessing patients for orthostatic hypotension both before and after treatment.
- Assessing patients for recent falls before each dialysis session.
- Securing power cords out of the walkway.
- Removing all clutter and avoiding placing items on the floor.
- Participating in staff education regarding the risk of falls.
- Helping to educate patients and family about fall prevention.
- Assisting patients to walk safely.
- Providing ready access to gait assistance devices.
- Using in-floor weight scales that are not elevated.
- Using proper body mechanics when transferring patients.
- Utilizing lift-equipment (such as the Hoyer lifts) instead of lifting patients manually.

> **Review Video: Fall Prevention**
> Visit mometrix.com/academy and enter code: 972452

VIOLENT AND AGGRESSIVE PATIENT BEHAVIOR

Violence and aggression may occur among patients or family members, posing a danger to others. Risk factors include mental health disorders, access to weapons, and history of personal or family violence, abuse, animal cruelty, fire setting, and/or substance abuse. Signs of impending danger from violence and aggression are as follows:

- **Violence** is a physical act perpetrated against an inanimate object, animal, or other person with the intent to cause harm. Violence often results from anger, frustration, or fear and occurs because the perpetrators believe that they are threatened or that their opinion is right and the other person is wrong. Violence may occur suddenly without warning or following aggressive behavior. Violence can result in death or severe injury if the individual attacks. The hemodialysis technician must back away and seek safety. Security should be called when safe to do so.
- **Aggression** is the communication of a threat or intended act of violence and will often occur before an act of violence. This communication can occur verbally or nonverbally. Gestures, shouting, speaking increasingly loudly, invasion of personal space, or prolonged eye contact are examples of aggression requiring the individual be redirected or removed from the situation. The hemodialysis technician should avoid prolonged direct eye contact.

ACTIVE SHOOTERS

The dialysis facility should have a plan in place for environmental emergencies, such as an active shooter. The plan should include risks, notification process, lockdown procedures, evacuation procedures, escape routes, and chain of command for emergency response. Staff members should practice and review the procedures at least every 6 months. Safety precautions, such as limiting access, requiring ID badges, and having panic buttons should be in place. In an active shooter situation, the goal is to minimize the loss of life, and the three courses of action that are available to the person include running, hiding, or fighting back. The choice depends on the situation and the time available. Active shooters also often use explosive devices (such as pipe bombs) as well as guns. If a shooter has not yet entered the unit, then those who can run and hide should likely do so, and doors should be locked and barricaded, but if the shooter is inside the room and shooting, then hiding may be useful if there are places to hide; otherwise, those present should arm themselves with whatever is available, such as equipment that can be thrown or fire extinguishers that can spray the perpetrator.

BOMB THREATS

If a dialysis center receives a bomb threat, the exact time the threat is received must be recorded and the way in which the threat was received. If by telephone, the person taking the call should try to stay calm and ask for as much information as possible (Where is it? What kind of bomb? Who are you? When will it explode? Why?) and record the person's exact words while trying to keep the person on the line and signaling to others to call security and 9-1-1. If a suspicious item (such as a package) is found, it should not be approached or touched, and the area around it should be immediately cleared. Emergency evacuation should be carried out utilizing emergency disconnect procedures (clamp, disconnect, and cap venous and arterial lines or use a clamp and cut kit). Ambulatory patients should be assisted first, then those who can walk with assistance, and last those who are non-ambulatory and need staff to place then in wheelchairs. Patients should be immediately directed toward the safest evacuation route and kept at a safe distance from the possible explosion.

DISASTER PREPARATION

CMS requirements for disaster preparation include developing a disaster plan, training staff at least annually in emergency procedures, developing safe evacuation plans as well as sheltering in place, training patients at least once a year on what to do in case of emergencies, teaching patients to self-disconnect, having a communication plan, planning and coordinating drills with local health care coalitions, displaying patient care staff CPR certification, and conducting disaster drills (large and small scale) at least once a year. Some states may require more frequent drills. Drills should include practice for all different types of possible disasters, both natural (tornados, hurricanes, flooding, fires) and man-made (bombs, shootings). Patients should be involved in disaster drills and should be taught evacuation routes and should practice emergency disconnect procedures. Procedures should be reviewed at least quarterly. Patients should be provided information about emergency backup centers as well as the 3-day emergency diet that should be utilized for those who must shelter in place and cannot access hemodialysis equipment.

FIRE SAFETY PROCEDURES

Fire drills should be carried out routinely (usually monthly). If a fire occurs on the dialysis unit, and the fire is small and contained, the first step should be to pull the fire alarm and to use a fire extinguisher from a distance of 8-10 feet (PASS procedure):

- **P**ull the retaining pin.
- **A**im at the base of the fire.

- **S**queeze the handle to discharge the agent.
- **S**weep from side to side.

Larger fires that cannot be controlled or extinguished with handheld extinguisher, cause excessive smoke, or trigger sprinklers require evacuation of staff and patients:

- Carry out emergency disconnect procedure for patients on dialysis: Clamp, disconnect, and cap venous and arterial lines or use a clamp and cut kit. Disconnect ambulatory patients first, those who can ambulate with assistance next, and those who are unable to ambulate last.
- Instruct ambulatory patients to evacuate according to protocol and help those who require assistance or wheelchair to exit as quickly as possible.
- Cover mouths and noses with damp cloths if smoke is severe.
- Close as many doors and windows as possible during evacuation to contain the fire.

LIFE SAFETY CODE REQUIREMENTS

The National Fire Protection Association publishes the Life Safety Code (AKA NFPA 101), which is a consensus standard to help to reduce danger to people from fires. While the standards themselves are not legally binding, they have been used as the basis for legal regulations at local, state, and national levels. CMS requires compliance with NFPA 101 standards in order to receive reimbursement for Medicare or Medicaid. A dialysis unit may be a free-standing facility, classified as having ambulatory health care occupancy. If the dialysis unit is part of an inpatient facility serving in-patients, it is classified as having health care occupancy. The LSC requirements under CMS include a provision for facilities to have a sprinkler system and central monitoring system although existing facilities that do not have sprinkler systems are grandfathered in. Facilities must have automatic notification-equipped fire detection and alarms. If states receive waiver from CMS, facilities in that state only have to meet state requirements. Each facility is required to have a disaster preparedness plan and to establish evacuation routes. Fire drills should be held periodically, but simulated patients and empty chairs rather than actual patients may be used for practice evacuations.

CDC GUIDELINES FOR SUPPLY SAFETY

CDC's recommendations regarding carrying supplies in pockets:

- The CDC recommends that dialysis **staff do not carry supplies in their pockets**. Needle caps come off very easily, and could injure the hemodialysis technician. Gloves, alcohol swabs, saline flushes and tape can be easily contaminated.
- Place glove boxes at designated locations throughout the unit to make them readily available to staff in a patient emergency.
- Tape should be used only once on one patient. Throw the remainder away at the end of each treatment.

The CDC's position was upheld in the *Medicare Coverage for ESRD Facilities* federal guideline changes. Infractions of the CDC's recommendations can result in Medicare citations if the surveyors find staff carrying supplies in their pockets during an accreditation survey.

PROFESSIONAL ETHICS AND BOUNDARIES

The hemodialysis technician must also always maintain high standards with regards to the following:

- **Professional ethics**: The hemodialysis technician should understand the duties of the position and all policies and procedures, should provide safe and effective care in keeping with the standards of the profession, and should treat all patients and co-workers with respect and consideration. The hemodialysis technician should be aware of the HIPAA regulations and respect the patients' right to privacy.
- **Professional boundaries**: The hemodialysis technician must remember that a patient is not the same as a family member or friend despite long-term relationships (in some cases) and should avoid sharing inappropriate personal information (such as telephone number, personal life details, or personal problems) or giving advice unrelated to treatment (such as about patient family problems). The hemodialysis technician should avoid all inappropriate touching or relationships, gift giving, and favors and should avoid discussion of or contact with patients on social media.

PATIENT RIGHTS

Patient rights relating to dialysis include the following:

- The patient has the right to be informed about the nature of the illness.
- The patient has the right to be informed about the treatment procedure and the risks involved.
- The patient must be informed regarding any possible treatment alternatives.
- The patient has the right to confidentiality and personal privacy.
- The patient must be allowed input into his or her treatment plan.
- An adult who is judged mentally competent has the right to refuse treatment.

A patient with certain health conditions may be excluded from dialysis. In some states, any person requiring dialysis is guaranteed dialysis should he or she desire the treatment, regardless of state of health. The US Renal Physicians Association has issued guidelines for stopping treatment or excluding a patient from treatment.

INFORMED CONSENT

Before any invasive procedure is performed on a patient, informed written consent must be obtained. Dialysis is categorized as an invasive procedure. In the case where a patient requires emergency dialysis and is unable to give informed written consent, the next of kin or an individual who holds a durable power of attorney may provide written consent on the patient's behalf. The consent form must indicate the nature of the procedure. The benefits, possible complications, risks, and alternatives to the treatment should be explained in the consent form. The form should indicate that the benefits, possible complications, risks, and alternative treatments have been discussed with the patient and were understood by the patient. The structure of the consent form depends on the facility and the facility's lawyer. Any significant change in procedure requires a new consent form. A separate consent form is required if access procedures are to be performed.

ADVANCED DIRECTIVES

An advanced directive is a legal document specifying the medical treatments that can be administered to an individual in the event he or she should become incapacitated. An advanced directive can take the form of a durable power of attorney or a living will. Different states have different requirements regarding advanced directives. The dialysis facility personnel should be familiar with the laws regarding advanced directives within their state. Patients have the right to refuse treatment regardless of the views of the facility personnel. Patients can refuse to begin or refuse to continue dialysis.

The Patient Self-Determination Act is a law enacted in 1991 that applies to healthcare organizations and healthcare providers. The law requires patients to be given information about their legal rights regarding medical treatment and their rights to refuse treatment.

ROLE OF THE PRECEPTOR

The dialysis technician is often in the position of having many roles in clinical practice, including educating others and serving as a **preceptor** for students who are studying to enter the field. While mentoring may entail a long-term relationship, preceptoring is usually a time-limited arrangement related to a term of study, such as a semester, orientation period, or a clinical rotation. The dialysis technician must balance responsibilities and ensure that he/she is able to provide adequate clinical supervision and guidance to the student on a daily basis. This may require coordinating schedules and planning carefully to ensure all responsibilities can be met. The preceptor helps the student to understand his/her impact on care, duties, and roles by including the student in all activities. The preceptor may engage in shared care as well as direct supervision in order to improve the student's skills.

TREATMENT MODALITIES

TRANSPLANT

Following a kidney transplant, a patient may require temporary dialysis to remove excess fluid, to treat an electrolyte imbalance, or to treat symptoms of uremia. Patients receiving renal and extrarenal transplants are given large amounts of fluid during the procedure to ensure cardiac stability. Hemofiltration is often necessary to remove the excess fluid that accumulated during surgery. In renal transplantation, function may not return to the transplanted kidney immediately. Renal transplant patients may experience acute rejection or acute tubular necrosis and require dialysis on a temporary basis. Extrarenal transplantation patients may also have renal disease or acute kidney injury. Techniques may be employed to treat the symptoms of renal disease or acute kidney injury.

ISSUES WITH DIALYZING A TRANSPLANT PATIENT

Internal bleeding is a concern for the first 24 hours following surgery. The patient's blood pressure should be monitored and hypotension reported to the physician. **Hypotension** can cause the transplanted kidney to become ischemic. The **surgical site** must be properly maintained. As **hemorrhage** and bleeding may occur after surgery, heparin-free dialysis should be utilized to keep anticoagulation to a minimum. It is common for a patient to experience **electrolyte imbalances** after transplantation. Hyperkalemia, an electrolyte imbalance, is often seen in transplant patients with impaired function of the organ. However, hyperkalemia can also be caused by immunosuppressants. There is also an increased **risk of infection** with the administration of immunosuppressants. Immediately after surgery, bacterial infections of the wound, urinary tract, and lungs are prevalent. Viral infections become more common in the weeks following surgery.

COMPLICATIONS OF DIALYSIS POST-TRANSPLANT

It is extremely important to maintain fluid balance in patients following a kidney transplant. If dialysis is needed by the post-transplant patient, extreme care should be taken not to cause hypotension by removing too much fluid. **Hypotension** could cause the transplanted kidney to become hypoperfused, which can result in organ failure. The patient who has received a kidney transplant has had major surgery. As a result, dialysis should be **heparin-free** to avoid causing bleeding at the surgery site. The patient may be **catabolic** due to steroid treatment. The **blood urea nitrogen may be high** compared to the creatinine level. The patient may be **hypertensive** as a result of steroid treatment. Steroid treatment also causes edema in the tissues. If the patient develops an infection or experiences organ rejection, then **hypoproteinemia** and edema will follow. **Cardiac dysrhythmias** and **pulmonary congestion** are to be expected.

HOME HEMODIALYSIS

Home hemodialysis can potentially be done by patients of all ages if they are properly trained. Patients should be informed of the possibility of home hemodialysis and assessed for suitability. **Assessment for suitability** is conducted by the multidisciplinary dialysis team. Medical, psychosocial, and vocational factors should be taken into consideration. The home itself should be inspected for suitability. The plumbing, water, and electricity must meet certain standards, and there must be adequate space for the equipment. Minor modifications to the home may be necessary. Contraindications for home hemodialysis include serious cardiovascular conditions, lack of adequate access, history of medical noncompliance, lack of aid at home, inability to learn the required technique, lack of motivation, and excessive anxiety.

Understand Quality-Related Issues

CQI AND TQM

CQI stands for **continuous quality improvement**. CQI involves the use of data collection and observation to improve outcomes. The data collected and observations are used to develop new methods and better approaches to achieve better outcomes. Through the use of CQI, caregivers can identify potential problem areas before difficulties arise. CQI can also be used to assess the relationship between cost and quality.

TQM stands for **total quality management**. This term refers to the willingness of all members of the dialysis facility to exceed minimum standards of performance. This is achieved through compliance with the regulatory requirements and the constant striving to improve patient care and outcomes. For CQI to work, TQM must be practiced by every member in the organization.

NATIONAL KIDNEY FOUNDATION: KIDNEY DISEASE OUTCOMES QUALITY INITIATIVE

The National Kidney Foundation-Kidney Disease Outcomes Quality Initiative (NKF-KDOQI) has established guidelines for the treatment of dialysis patients. These guidelines are meant to improve care and outcome. The guidelines are clinical practice guidelines and are evidence-based. There are 13 different sets of guidelines dealing with different aspects of chronic kidney disease and dialysis treatment. These guidelines discuss diabetes, anemia, nutrition, hemodialysis adequacy, peritoneal dialysis adequacy, vascular access, chronic kidney disease, bone metabolism and bone disease, cardiovascular disease, Hepatitis C, kidney transplant, glomerulonephritis, and acute kidney injury. These guidelines are widely accepted in the United States, and have also been translated to other languages.

MEDICARE'S COP FOR THE DIALYSIS FACILITY'S PHYSICAL ENVIRONMENT

Medicare addressed four areas in its new Conditions of Participation *(CoP)*:

- **Facility building safety**: The building must comply with the 2000 guidelines of the National Fire Protection Association.
- **Equipment maintenance**: All equipment in the unit must be maintained per the manufacturer's recommendations.

- **Emergency preparedness and fire safety**: Both staff *and* patients must have emergency preparedness training. Emergency equipment must be available in the dialysis facility, such as oxygen, airways, a suction defibrillator, emergency drugs, and fire extinguishers.
- **The patient care environment**: Dialysis units must maintain a temperature in the treatment area that is comfortable for the general patient population, and must make provisions for those patients who are uncomfortable. Patients may bring their own blankets or the facility may provide them, but access sites may not be covered from view by the staff.

STORAGE OF MEDICATIONS, EQUIPMENT AND SUPPLIES

Storage considerations on the dialysis unit:

- **Dialysis medications**: Must be kept in locked cart, cabinet, or container and maintained at the correct temperature (frozen below -5 °C, cold storage at no more than 8 °C, cool at 8-15 °C, and room temperature at 20-25 °C). Crash carts must be stored in a secure area. Medication carts may be unlocked when they are under direct supervision of staff members. Concentrated electrolytes must be stored separately from other drugs. All IV bags that are stored must be labeled with the expiration date.
- **Equipment and supplies**: Clean and dirty equipment and supplies must be stored in separate areas, and reprocessed dialyzers must be stored separately from new dialyzers. Supplies may not be placed on the floor but on shelving or in cabinets. Safety data sheets must be available for all stored hazardous chemicals. Items must be stored at least 18 inches below sprinkler head or 24 inches below the ceiling if there is no sprinkler system. Supplies must be stored at least 6 inches above the floor.

ORGANIZATION OF THE DIALYSIS FACILITY

The **medical director** of a dialysis facility oversees the medical care of the patients. Every facility providing dialysis has written policies and procedures designed to guide patient care and clinical practice. These policies and procedures govern the quality of care, upkeep and use of equipment, and medical procedure protocols. The Joint Commission, which governs special care units, requires that policies be written by the dialysis team and approved by the facility's administrators. The Joint Commission does not control the functioning of freestanding dialysis facilities. The policies and procedures of freestanding facilities are determined by the governing body of the individual facility. The governing body is comprised of the medical director, nursing director, and facility administrator. The policies and procedures of freestanding facilities must adhere to state laws and the rules of the Centers for Medicare and Medicaid Services (CMS).

Communication Skills with Staff Members

PERSONNEL INVOLVED IN THE TREATMENT OF A DIALYSIS PATIENT

Dialysis treatment involves a number of different types of healthcare professionals. The team members involved in the treatment of a dialysis patient may include physicians, nurses, medical technicians, dietitians, psychologists, and pharmacists. Furthermore, it may be necessary to involve social workers and rehabilitation counselors. The members of the dialysis team work together to ensure the best possible patient care. Family members also play an important role in the treatment of the dialysis patient.

NEPHROLOGIST

Nephrology is a field of medicine concerned with the anatomy and function of the kidney and the diagnosis and treatment of kidney disease. The nephrologist is responsible for deciding when the patient has developed end-stage renal disease (ESRD) and when dialysis is necessary. A nephrologist is a physician with a specialization in internal medicine that has undertaken additional training in nephrology. Individuals with chronic kidney disease should be seen by a nephrologist, as soon as possible upon diagnosis, prior to the development of ESRD. Early medical care by a nephrologist may improve or maintain the patient's kidney function and delay the patient's need for dialysis. The nephrologist determines when dialysis must be initiated and writes the dialysis prescription.

DIALYSIS NURSE

Nurses in a dialysis facility are responsible for the care of the patients and supervise the technicians who perform the dialysis procedure. The nurses are also responsible for educating the patient and the patient's family, for providing patient support, and for assessing the patient on a continual basis. The nurse is typically responsible for organizing any necessary multidisciplinary case conferences to deal with issues regarding the patient's health or well-being. Different types of dialysis units may have different models of organization. In facilities using a primary nursing model, each patient is assigned a primary nurse who oversees his or her care. Dialysis facilities may also use the case-management model. The case-management model is designed to provide continuity of care. This model may involve providing care not only in the dialysis unit, but in outpatient facilities and in the patient's home.

QUALITIES NECESSARY

While the exact requirements for working as a dialysis nurse vary depending on regulations of the facility, all facilities have certain requirements:

- A dialysis nurse is required to be a professional nurse and to have at least one year of medical-surgical nursing.
- The nurse must be licensed to practice in the state in question.
- Certification in a related specialty, such as nephrology or critical care, is desirable.
- Experience working in a critical care situation or emergency department can be valuable.
- Dialysis facilities generally have a training program for newly hired and inexperienced nurses.
- A dialysis nurse is often required to teach patients, family members, coworkers, and other healthcare professionals about dialysis.
- Patience and an ability to teach are essential characteristics for a dialysis nurse.
- The dialysis nurse must be able to delegate assignments and evaluate the care given to patients by other healthcare workers.

ADVANCED PRACTICE NURSE

There are an increasing number of advanced practice nurses (APNs) working in dialysis facilities. An APN working in a dialysis facility may be a nurse practitioner or a clinical nurse specialist. APNs work in all aspects of renal care and work in different types of healthcare facilities. An APN is trained to manage the care of patients in all stages of renal disease. The number of individuals with chronic kidney disease is increasing, and the number of nephrologists available to treat these patients is decreasing. A shortage of nephrologists has been predicted. APNs can help provide necessary patient care that would otherwise be lacking.

DIALYSIS TECHNICIAN

A technician in a dialysis unit must be knowledgeable about the principles of mechanics and physics. An understanding of computer technology is needed. Technicians working in the area of patient care need a basic knowledge of human anatomy and physiology. A background in the pathophysiology of renal disease is required. The technician working in patient care needs to understand the principles and theories related to dialysis, the complications that may arise from dialysis treatment, and how to ensure the health of the vascular space. Although technicians are supervised by nursing staff, the technician who is working with a patient needs to be able to monitor patient response and make clinical judgments about the health of the patient. Dialysis technicians are regulated by the state, which may require licensure, registration, or certification. State regulations for practice vary.

DUTIES

The duties of a dialysis technician in a dialysis facility vary depending on the state. Different states have different regulations. Dialysis technicians do fulfill 2 important roles. One of these roles involves assembling and maintaining equipment. The dialysis equipment must be maintained on a regular basis. Technicians qualified to care for the expensive equipment are a valuable part of the team. Technicians may also be directly involved in patient care. In this case, the technician works under the supervision of the nurses in the facility. Technicians may be involved in both equipment maintenance and patient care. Technicians in a dialysis facility work as a member of the team to ensure quality patient care.

RENAL DIETITIAN

The renal dietitian helps to manage the patient's diet through all stages of renal disease. An appropriate diet can delay the need for dialysis. After the patient has started dialysis, nutritional status should be monitored. An appropriate diet for a patient depends on a number of factors. The renal dietitian works with the patient, the patient's family, the nurses, the dialysis technicians, the physicians, and the social workers. The dietitian assesses the patient's dietary needs and monitors the patient's condition on an ongoing basis. The patient's diet is reevaluated as necessary. The dietitian provides information to the patient and his or her family about the requirements of the diet and the need to adhere to the diet.

SOCIAL WORKER

A patient with renal disease may require psychosocial support throughout his or her illness. The Council of Nephrology Social Workers has defined two major goals for nephrology social workers. These include promoting awareness regarding the psychosocial problems experienced by patients with kidney disease, and developing methods to treat these problems. The job of the renal social worker is to help the patient and his or her family adapt to the situation and the requirements of treatment. The renal social worker consults with the patient, the patient's family, and the other team members in the dialysis facility. The renal social worker must be licensed if required by the state in which he or she is practicing.

VERBAL AND NONVERBAL COMMUNICATION

Effective communication includes:

- **Verbal aspects**: It's important to begin communication with an introduction and greeting. Open-ended questions are likely to promote better communication than yes/no questions. The hemodialysis technician should be honest in all communications and demonstrate a willingness to listen to and collaborate with others, should encourage others to participate in conversations, ask for clarification when needed, make observations ("You are shaking") rather than judgments ("You seem afraid"), and indicate reality without challenging misperceptions. The hemodialysis technician should also respect the right of others to end communication.

- **Nonverbal aspects**: This includes practicing active listening to show interest in what others have to say, nodding the head, maintaining appropriate eye contact (recognizing that some cultural groups use eye contact differently), turning toward individuals who are speaking, using a soothing tone of voice, maintaining the appropriate distance and respecting personal space, and avoiding the appearance of being rushed.

BARRIERS TO THERAPEUTIC COMMUNICATION

Barriers to therapeutic communication includes:

- Actions and attitudes:
  - Failing to engage with others or to indicate interest in their opinions.
  - Making negative judgments or devaluing others' feelings.
  - Openly disagreeing with others or changing the subject.
  - Taking a defensive attitude toward any criticism.
  - Providing unwanted and/or unsolicited advice.
  - Monopolizing conversations and not allowing others to speak.

- Physical barriers/conditions:
  - Closed doors, physically-separated work area.
  - Environmental impediments, such as noise, poor lighting.
  - Hearing impairment (deaf, wearing hearing aids).
  - Impaired speech (post-stroke, neurological disorders).

- Cultural/Language differences:
  - Failure to recognize differences in communication approaches, including both verbal and nonverbal behaviors (eye contact, gestures, turn-taking).
  - Difference in gender roles may make some patients uncomfortable.
  - Patients may speak no or little English, and translators may not be readily available.

CHT Practice Test

Want to take this practice test in an online interactive format?
Check out the bonus page, which includes interactive practice questions and
much more: **https://www.mometrix.com/bonus948/certhemotech**

1. Peritoneal dialysis (PD) differs from hemodialysis in which of the following ways?

- a. PD requires both vascular access and abdominal access
- b. PD cannot be done at home
- c. PD access is by an intra-abdominal catheter
- d. Sterile dialysate is not required for PD

2. The main difference between an arteriovenous shunt (AVS) and an arteriovenous fistula (AVF) is an:

- a. AVS is entirely within the arm.
- b. AVF is entirely within the arm.
- c. AVF is more likely to become clotted or infected.
- d. AVF requires an external tube.

3. Which of the following dialyzers is used currently?

- a. Kiil
- b. Flat plate
- c. Coil
- d. Hollow tube

4. Which of the following kidney structures connects with and delivers urine directly to the ureter?

- a. Pelvis
- b. Calyx
- c. Glomerulus
- d. Cortex

5. The glomerular filtration rate is an important index of renal function and in the normal adult is approximately:

- a. $50 \text{ mL/min/1.73 m}^2$.
- b. $75 \text{ mL/min/1.73 m}^2$.
- c. $125 \text{ mL/min/1.73 m}^2$.
- d. $200 \text{ mL/min/1.73 m}^2$.

6. All of the following substances are produced by the kidney EXCEPT:

- a. renin.
- b. aldosterone.
- c. erythropoietin.
- d. calcitriol.

7. The most likely cause of post–renal failure is:

a. severe dehydration.
b. nephrotoxic drug.
c. glomerulonephritis.
d. benign prostatic hypertrophy.

8. The most common cause of chronic kidney disease in the United States is:

a. diabetes.
b. hypertension.
c. glomerulonephritis.
d. polycystic kidney disease.

9. Which of the following conditions is LEAST likely to be caused by uremia?

a. Itching
b. Edema (swelling) of the extremities
c. Anemia
d. Urinary tract infection

10. All of following conditions are associated with chronic kidney failure EXCEPT:

a. low hemoglobin.
b. hypoparathyroidism.
c. hyperkalemia.
d. hyperphosphatemia.

11. What percentage of transplanted kidneys are functional 1 year after transplantation?

a. 90%
b. 70%
c. 50%
d. 30%

12. Which hemodialysis schedule is likely to be most efficient?

a. In-center hemodialysis, 3–4 hours a session, 3 days a week
b. Conventional home hemodialysis
c. Short daily home hemodialysis, 2–3 hours a session, 5–7 days a week
d. Nocturnal home hemodialysis, 8 hours during sleep, 3 days a week

13. The fluid restriction for most patients undergoing in-center hemodialysis is equal to urine volume/day plus:

a. 0 L.
b. 0.5 L.
c. 1 L.
d. 2 L.

14. Failure to excrete beta$_2$-microglobulin in patients with kidney failure predisposes the patient to:

a. pericarditis.
b. amyloidosis.
c. neuropathy.
d. seizures.

15. Blood tests for ferritin are performed in hemodialysis patients:

   a. to check for iron stores.
   b. to check for magnesium levels.
   c. as an alternative to hemoglobin concentration.
   d. to maintain electrolyte balance.

16. Which of the following phosphate binders would best control hyperphosphatemia with the fewest side effects in patients with end stage kidney disease?

   a. Aluminum hydroxide
   b. Calcium carbonate
   c. High dairy product diet
   d. Lanthanum carbonate

17. Hemodialysis patients should be taught to:

   a. put in their own needles.
   b. weigh themselves and record it.
   c. check their dialyzer settings and dialysate.
   d. do all of the above.

18. All of the following statements about vitamins in dialysis patients are true EXCEPT:

   a. dialysis does not remove water-soluble vitamins.
   b. supplemental B-complex vitamins should be given.
   c. vitamin D should be given to most dialysis patients.
   d. megadose fat- or water-soluble vitamins should not be given.

19. Osmosis is best defined as:

   a. diffusion of solute through a semipermeable membrane from a high- to low-solute concentration.
   b. diffusion of solvent through a semipermeable membrane from low- to high-solute concentration.
   c. a version of hydraulic pressure used in dialysis.
   d. diffusion of solvent through a semipermeable membrane from high- to low-solute concentration.

20. In hemodialysis, blood and dialysate have which of the following properties?

   a. They flow in the same direction
   b. They flow in opposite directions
   c. They mix within the dialyzer
   d. They do not require a semipermeable membrane

21. In the dialyzer, water may be removed from:

   a. the intracellular compartment.
   b. the intravascular compartment.
   c. the interstitial compartment.
   d. all of the above compartments.

22. **Which site in the hemodialysis pathway has the highest positive pressure?**
    a. Arterial blood in the afferent tubing
    b. Blood entering the dialyzer fibers
    c. Blood leaving the dialyzer fibers
    d. Blood in the venous return

23. **The term "sieving coefficient of a membrane" refers to the:**
    a. fraction of solute that passes through the membrane by convection.
    b. amount of water required for solute drag through the membrane.
    c. concentration of pores in the membrane.
    d. size of the pores in the membrane.

24. **Water moves from one body compartment to another by:**
    a. ultrafiltration.
    b. active transport.
    c. osmotic forces.
    d. all of the above.

25. **Biocompatibility is best illustrated by:**
    a. synthetic membranes that do not adsorb blood proteins as well as cellulose membranes.
    b. independence from protein adsorption of the membrane.
    c. reprocessed dialyzers that have a lower biocompatibility than new ones.
    d. reprocessed dialyzers that have a better biocompatibility than new ones.

26. **The amount of fluid to be taken from the patient during hemodialysis:**
    a. is independent of the filtration pressure.
    b. requires the dialysate to have a higher pressure than the blood.
    c. may be calculated by subtracting the patient's estimated dry weight from the pre-dialysis weight and adding any fluid the patient receives during treatment.
    d. may be calculated by adding the patient's pre-dialysis weight and the amount of fluid the patient receives during treatment.

27. **The ultrafiltration coefficient of a dialyzer refers to the:**
    a. fluid that passes through the membrane in 1 hour.
    b. pressure in the blood compartment needed to force fluid through the membrane.
    c. pressure difference across the membrane.
    d. fluid that passes through the membrane in 1 minute.

28. **The molecular weight cutoff of a dialyzer is 12,000 daltons. Which of the following molecules would not pass through the membrane into the dialysate?**
    a. Phosphate
    b. Urea
    c. Albumin
    d. Sodium

29. Clearance of low-molecular-weight molecules by dialysis is accomplished mostly by:

    a. convection.
    b. diffusion.
    c. adsorption.
    d. solvent drag.

30. A hollow fiber dialyzer has which of the following properties?

    a. Very fine fiber tubes held in place by polyurethane material
    b. Fibers about 1 cm in width
    c. A high-membrane compliance
    d. A high resistance in the fibers, enhancing ultrafiltration pressure

31. Synthetic membranes have which of the following properties?

    a. They are cellulose membranes in which hydroxyl groups are replaced with acetate
    b. They have thick fiber walls
    c. They have poor adsorption
    d. They remove solute by diffusion only

32. If a dialyzer has a urea clearance rate (K) of 200 mL/min and a blood flow rate (Qb) of 300 mL/min, what volume of the blood will be cleared of urea in 1 minute?

    a. 100 mL
    b. 200 mL
    c. 300 mL
    d. 500 mL

33. To determine the most accurate clearance rate of a particular solute, one should:

    a. use water instead of blood.
    b. use a large-molecular-weight molecule.
    c. reduce the manufacturer's stated rate by 10%.
    d. measure the solute concentrations of blood going into and out of the dialyzer.

34. All of the following substances are added to the dialysate EXCEPT:

    a. bicarbonate.
    b. chloride.
    c. sodium.
    d. phosphate.

35. Sodium modeling refers to:

    a. changing the concentration of the dialysate sodium during the course of dialysis.
    b. injecting sodium chloride directly into the patient's vein.
    c. adjusting the sodium concentrate of the dialysate with normal saline.
    d. none of the above.

36. Conductivity is best defined as:

    a. a method of checking electrolyte levels in the dialysate.
    b. the voltage required to maintain the dialysis pump to achieve a given flow rate.
    c. a monitor and alarm system to measure dialysate flow rate.
    d. something that is measured once to check the final ionic concentrations of the dialysate.

37. Which of the following statements about the proportioning system is correct?

a. The concentrates are mixed manually
b. It relies on a continuous supply of fresh concentrate and treated water
c. The concentrates are heated after mixing
d. Fixed-ratio mixing is the only method used

38. An advantage of high-flux dialysis is:

a. small pore size.
b. fast removal of fluid.
c. retention of beta2-microglobulin in the blood.
d. slow blood flow, leading to more efficient removal of toxic substances.

39. A disadvantage of high-flux dialysis is:

a. acetate must be used instead bicarbonate buffer.
b. membrane biocompatibility is reduced.
c. pyrogen reactions are common.
d. post-dialysis fatigue is common.

40. All of the following statements regarding home dialysis are true EXCEPT:

a. a spouse's or other family member's assistance is desirable.
b. a visiting dialysis nurse may be employed.
c. the patient and assistant must train for 6–8 weeks.
d. it cannot be done during sleep.

41. In most dialysate systems, the temperature:

a. is maintained by a thermistor-controlled heater.
b. is maintained between 41–43 degrees Celsius.
c. of water is raised only after mixing with concentrate.
d. is decreased to increase diffusion.

42. Dialysate flow rate has which of the following properties?

a. Lower flow rates improve dialysate efficiency
b. It is always preset
c. It may vary from 0–2000 mL/min
d. Low water pressure may set off an alarm

43. Which of the following statements about blood leaks in the dialysis system is correct?

a. They require more than 10 mL of blood to trigger an alarm
b. They are detected by use of a light source and photocell
c. The blood can be returned to the patient
d. They cannot be differentiated from false alarms

44. Dialysate pH is kept in which of the following ranges?

a. 7.0–7.4
b. 7.35–7.45
c. 6.0–7.0
d. 8.0–9.0

45. **Which of the following statements about fluid removal from the blood is correct?**
    a. It is achieved with a higher dialysate pressure than blood pressure
    b. It depends on the transmembrane pressure (TMP)
    c. It requires that the TMP must be calculated mathematically by the technician
    d. The manufacturer's ultrafiltration constant is usually lower than the true value

46. **Dialysis machines control the rate of fluid removal by:**
    a. volume control.
    b. flow control.
    c. either volume or flow control.
    d. neither volume nor flow control.

47. **Drip chambers in the extracorporeal circulation do all the following EXCEPT:**
    a. monitor arterial and venous pressure by attached gauges.
    b. trap air.
    c. prevent blood clots from reaching the patient.
    d. pump blood into the dialyzer.

48. **Which of the following statements about extracorporeal circulation is correct?**
    a. Approximately 100–250 mL are outside the patient's body at any time
    b. The arterial tubing is blue, and the venous tubing is red
    c. A heparin infusion line is connected to the tubing at the venous exit
    d. All blood tubing is manufactured to the same national standard

49. **Which of the following statements about transducer protectors is correct?**
    a. They measure arterial pressure only
    b. They measure venous pressure only
    c. They use membranes with a pore size of 1.0 micron
    d. They use hydrophobic membranes to keep fluid from passing through

50. **Blood flow into the dialyzer is usually:**
    a. controlled by a piston type pump.
    b. inversely proportional to the pump speed.
    c. limited to less than 250 mL/min.
    d. done by manual hand cranking.

51. **Which pressure in the dialysis circuit is usually negative?**
    a. Arterial pressure
    b. Pre-dialyzer pressure
    c. Post-dialyzer pressure
    d. Venous pressure

52. **Which of the following will set off the pre-pump high-pressure alarm?**
    a. An increase in the blood pump speed
    b. Kinking of the arterial bloodline
    c. A decrease in the blood pump speed
    d. Infiltration of the arterial needle

53. A low-pressure alarm in the venous (post-dialyzer) line is likely to be set off by:

    a. a blockage in the blood tubing between the monitoring site and the venous needle.
    b. an infiltration of the venous needle.
    c. a clot in the venous access.
    d. a blockage in the blood tubing before the monitoring site.

54. Which of the following statements about an air detector is correct?

    a. It is present in the pre-dialyzer blood tubing
    b. It uses an ultrasonic device to detect air in the blood path
    c. It sets off an alarm and clamps the pre-dialyzer blood tubing
    d. All of the above statements are correct

55. How is the anticoagulant heparin given during the dialysis treatment?

    a. Intermittently
    b. As a single bolus
    c. By continuous infusion
    d. By all of the above ways

56. A sorbent is best described as a:

    a. material that moisturizes the dialysis membrane.
    b. material that is added to the dialysate to buffer it and keep the pH constant.
    c. continuous dialysate disinfection system that removes bacteria and endotoxins.
    d. type of electronic device that measures blood pressure.

57. Which of the following statements about sorbent dialysis is correct?

    a. It needs a continuous supply of fresh water to add to new dialysate
    b. In preparing the dialysate, 6 liters of water are added to premixed chemicals
    c. The duration of the dialysis procedure cannot be altered
    d. It requires a six-layered cartridge

58. Which type of arteriovenous fistula is likely to result in high blood flow with the fewest complications?

    a. Artery side to vein side
    b. Artery side to vein end
    c. Artery end to vein side
    d. Artery end to vein end

59. For which type of dialysis patient is a central venous catheter blood access appropriate?

    a. A patient waiting for a fistula to mature
    b. A patient with acute renal failure
    c. A patient waiting for a peritoneal dialysis catheter
    d. All of the above patients

60. Which of the following statements about arteriovenous grafts is correct?

    a. They are more prone to thrombosis than arteriovenous fistulae.
    b. They are less prone to cause stenosis than arteriovenous fistulae.
    c. They are less prone to infection than arteriovenous fistulae.
    d. They have a longer lifespan than arteriovenous fistulae.

61. **Care of a new arteriovenous fistula should include all of the following EXCEPT:**
    a. checking for redness, purulent discharge, or other signs of infection.
    b. being certain the surgical incision is well healed.
    c. cannulating the vessel to see if the blood flow is adequate.
    d. listening for a bruit and feeling for a thrill at the fistula site.

62. **An antiseptic that kills bacteria when wet is:**
    a. 70% alcohol.
    b. 10% povidone iodine (Betadine).
    c. chlorhexidine gluconate with 70% alcohol (ChloraPrep).
    d. sodium hypochlorite (Except Plus).

63. **Which of the following arteries is most commonly used for an arteriovenous fistula?**
    a. Ulnar artery
    b. Radial artery
    c. Brachial artery
    d. Femoral artery

64. **The hemodialysis technician who is about to insert a needle into the arteriovenous fistula should first do all of the following EXCEPT:**
    a. feel for flat spots and check for a thrill.
    b. listen for a bruit.
    c. place the needle into a previous cannulation spot.
    d. check skin temperature.

65. **During needle insertion, it is important for the hemodialysis technician to always:**
    a. keep the bevel facing down.
    b. rotate the needle 180 degrees after insertion.
    c. cannulate the venous access in an antegrade manner (with the blood flow).
    d. cannulate the venous access in a retrograde manner (against the blood flow).

66. **Using the buttonhole technique for blood access, the technician should:**
    a. use a sharp followed by a blunt needle.
    b. only use a sharp needle.
    c. insert arterial and venous needles in a retrograde direction.
    d. leave an old scab in place.

67. **To diminish vasovagal reactions and needle phobia in the dialysis patient, the technician should ask the patient to:**
    a. lie down in a recumbent position.
    b. tense the muscles in the nonaccess hand for 10–20 seconds during needle insertion.
    c. cannulate his or her own vessels.
    d. do all of the above.

68. **Recirculation refers to:**
    a. recycling used dialysate into fresh dialysate.
    b. mixing dialyzed venous blood with blood entering the arterial needle.
    c. bypassing the fistula via collateral vessels.
    d. none of the above.

69. A diabetic patient undergoing dialysis complains of tingling, numbness, and cold in the hand below the access site. The most likely cause is:

a. steal syndrome.
b. recirculation.
c. infiltration.
d. an aneurysm.

70. Common sites of stenosis in patients with an arteriovenous fistula include all the following EXCEPT:

a. the vein next to the anastomosis.
b. along the outflow vein
c. the large draining vein of the arm near the shoulder.
d. the artery next to the anastomosis.

71. A thrombosis is LEAST likely to develop with which of the following vascular access methods?

a. A central venous catheter
b. An arteriovenous graft
c. An arteriovenous fistula
d. All of the above

72. High-output cardiac failure is a complication of arteriovenous fistula or grafting. All of the following actions are a part of this condition EXCEPT:

a. increased venous return to the heart.
b. decreased cardiac workload.
c. reduced resistance in the arterial bed.
d. activation of the renin–angiotensin system.

73. Which of the following statements about grafts used for arteriovenous shunts for dialysis patients is correct?

a. They cannot be made from human or animal blood vessels
b. They can be made from collagen or expanded polytetrafluoroethylene
c. They take longer to mature than fistulas
d. They have a lower rate of clotting than fistulas

74. When placing a needle into a graft, a hemodialysis technician may do which of the following?

a. Use three sides to cannulate the graft, not just the top
b. Cannulate at the junction of the graft with the native vessel
c. Keep arterial and venous needles less than 1 inch apart
d. Place both arterial and venous needles in a retrograde (against direction of blood flow) manner

75. Which of the following veins is most suitable for hemodialysis catheter placement?

a. Subclavian
b. Femoral
c. Right internal jugular
d. Left internal jugular

M⊘metrix

76. **To prevent infection in catheters, hemodialysis technicians should be sure to:**
    a. wash hands and use sterile gloves.
    b. wear a mask, and ask the patient to wear a mask as well.
    c. remove wet dressing, dry around the site, and replace with fresh dressing,
    d. do all of the above.

77. **When the low-pressure alarm rings, signaling inadequate flow, the technician should be sure to:**
    a. reset the pressure alarm.
    b. switch arterial and venous lines.
    c. flush the catheter with saline.
    d. give a thrombolytic enzyme through the catheter.

78. **An advantage of catheter and port catheter devices is:**
    a. they are less likely than fistulas to become infected.
    b. they have higher blood flows over time.
    c. needle entry is not required.
    d. they are less apt to induce clotting.

79. **A heavyset patient arrives for dialysis in a wheelchair. He has difficulty standing without assistance. Which technique would be most appropriate to transfer him to the dialysis chair?**
    a. Portable lift device
    b. Slide board
    c. Stand and pivot
    d. Simple three person lift

80. **If a small fire breaks out in the dialysis center, which of the following safety sequences is correct?**
    a. Contain the fire, activate the alarm, and rescue the patients
    b. Disconnect patients from the machines, and first evacuate patients who cannot walk
    c. When using a fire extinguisher, pull the pin, aim the nozzle at the base of the flames, squeeze the handle, and spray from side to side at the base of the flames
    d. Give all patients and staff respirator masks, and await the fire department

81. **Using sterile technique, a hemodialysis technician should avoid all the following EXCEPT:**
    a. touching the needle to the outside of a saline bag before penetrating the port.
    b. touching the heparin syringe tip or the end of the heparin line.
    c. getting the sterile packet wet.
    d. washing hands and using sterile gloves.

82. **Use of protective equipment and techniques are intended to protect patients and staff members. Examples include all of the following EXCEPT:**
    a. changing gloves between patients.
    b. wearing a gown to avoid contamination with splash or spray.
    c. always recapping used needles.
    d. wearing a face shield when injecting into blood lines.

146

Copyright © Mometrix Media. You have been licensed one copy of this document for personal use only. Any other reproduction or redistribution is strictly prohibited. All rights reserved.
This content is provided for test preparation purposes only and does not imply an endorsement by Mometrix of any particular political, scientific, or religious point of view.

83. Which of the following pathogens is most likely to be spread during dialysis treatment?

    a. Hepatitis B
    b. Hepatitis C
    c. Human immunodeficiency virus
    d. Tuberculosis

84. Which of the following should be avoided when drawing up medication into a syringe?

    a. Reading the drug name and concentration before drawing it up and then checking it twice
    b. Injecting air from the syringe into the vial equal to the amount of planned withdrawal
    c. Changing needles after half the volume is drawn up
    d. Expelling air bubbles from the syringe before injecting the contents

85. Correct statements concerning the charting of patient data include all of the following EXCEPT:

    a. each entry must be followed by the writer's name and title.
    b. entries must be printed for legibility.
    c. approved abbreviations may be used.
    d. errors must have a line through them, marked error, and initialed.

86. After a treatment, a patient below dry weight may have:

    a. edema.
    b. high blood pressure.
    c. dyspnea (shortness of breath).
    d. muscle cramping.

87. Which of the following alarms must be checked before dialysis begins?

    a. Blood leak detector
    b. Conductivity alarm
    c. The pH alarm
    d. All of the above alarms

88. In a patient with a fistula in one arm and an intravenous line in the other, manual blood pressure should be taken in the:

    a. arm above the intravenous line.
    b. arm above the fistula.
    c. leg with the patient supine.
    d. leg with the patient standing.

89. Which of the following vital signs is abnormal before dialysis in a 30-year-old male patient?

    a. Blood pressure: 145/95 mm Hg
    b. Pulse: 90/min and regular
    c. Temperature: 98.6o F (37oC)
    d. Respirations: 16/min

90. To calculate the amount of fluid removal from the patient during dialysis, all of the following values are used EXCEPT:

    a.   priming saline volume.
    b.   saline rinse back.
    c.   dietary intake.
    d.   volume of urine output.

91. When drawing blood samples for laboratory testing, the hemodialysis technician should draw samples:

    a.   after giving saline and heparin.
    b.   from the arterial blood line injection port.
    c.   into tubes with anticoagulant first.
    d.   and keep them on a warm surface.

92. The urea reduction ratio has which of the following properties?

    a.   It requires measurement of both pre- and post-dialysis blood urea nitrogen
    b.   It accounts for the production of urea during dialysis
    c.   It allows calculation of the time needed for dialysis
    d.   It allows calculation of urea removed by ultrafiltration

93. What is the urea kinetic modeling calculation?

    a.   It gives the minimum delivered dose
    b.   It gives the minimum prescribed dose
    c.   It gives both minimum delivered and prescribed doses
    d.   It is independent of dialyzer type

94. Which of the following statements is accurate with regards to priming the reprocessed dialyzer?

    a.   Priming the reprocessed dialyzer is done using Lactated Ringers solution.
    b.   Priming is critical to ensure air is removed from the venous line prior to attachment.
    c.   Priming should be done at low pump speed.
    d.   Testing for germicide should be done prior to priming

95. A dialysis patient has a history of heparin-induced thrombocytopenia (low platelets) and severe bleeding. What would be a good method of performing dialysis safely?

    a.   Skip the bolus dose of heparin, and give the infusion at a lower dose rate
    b.   Increase the time between bolus doses of heparin
    c.   Substitute warfarin for heparin
    d.   Use a regional citrate technique

96. A dialysis patient develops a purulent discharge at the exit site of a central catheter. Which of the following pathogens is the most likely to be cultured?

    a.   *Staphylococcus aureus*
    b.   *Clostridioides difficile*
    c.   *Enterococcus*
    d.   *Mycoplasma*

97. A hemodialysis patient suddenly develops trouble breathing, hives, itching, and hypotension. The most likely cause is:
   a. an air embolism.
   b. an anaphylactic reaction.
   c. angina.
   d. disequilibrium syndrome.

98. A patient undergoing hemodialysis complains of muscle cramps in the calves and feet. All of the following are likely causes EXCEPT:
   a. hypernatremia (high-sodium level).
   b. excess fluid removal.
   c. hypercalcemia (high-calcium level).
   d. hypokalemia (low potassium).

99. Which of the following may cause hemolysis of red blood cells during dialysis?
   a. Kinked blood lines
   b. Warm dialysis fluid
   c. Inadequate water treatment
   d. All of the above

100. For centers that reuse dialyzers, reprocessing includes:
   a. cleaning the bloodlines with heparinized saline.
   b. removing and warming the dialyzer.
   c. disinfecting the clamps and the outside of the dialysis machine.
   d. using chemical disinfectant or cold saline to disinfect the dialysate pathway.

101. Which of the following statements about the "first-use syndrome" is correct?
   a. It may be reduced by repeated rinsing of the dialyzer
   b. It is less common in dialyzers treated with ethylene oxide
   c. Both a and b are true
   d. Neither a nor b are true

102. Which of the following statements about preprocessing dialyzers is correct?
   a. It must be done manually
   b. It can be done manually or by machine
   c. It may be done on all commercial dialyzers
   d. It may be done according to the local center's protocol

103. Which of the following statements about new dialyzers is correct?
   a. They should not be preprocessed
   b. The total cell volume (TCV) does not need checking until after reprocessing
   c. They may be preprocessed to reduce noxious chemicals or materials
   d. The TCV needs to be checked against other dialyzers after reprocessing

104. At the end of treatment, which of the following actions should be done first?
   a. Blood rinse back
   b. Preclean the dialyzer
   c. Blood leak test
   d. Measure the dialyzer's total cell volume

105. Grounds for discarding a dialyzer include which of the following?

    a. The total cell volume is 85% of the original

    b. It has been exposed to more than one germicide

    c. Clearance is only 95%

    d. A few residual streaks of blood are seen on inspection

106. Which of the following germicides is most commonly used to disinfect dialyzers in the United States?

    a. Formaldehyde

    b. Glutaraldehyde

    c. Heat with citric acid

    d. Peracetic acid

107. What is an endotoxin?

    a. It is a germicide

    b. It is not adsorbed by dialysis membranes

    c. It is a toxin produced by certain bacteria

    d. It is a substance that is not harmful to the patient

108. Federal regulations require a center that reuses dialyzers to have:

    a. a system of quality assurance.

    b. a system of quality control.

    c. both a and b.

    d. neither a nor b.

109. Which of the following substances is the most common impurity in tap water?

    a. Sodium chloride

    b. Carbonic acid

    c. Calcium nitrate

    d. Calcium carbonate

110. The average hemodialysis patient is exposed to how many liters of water a week?

    a. 10 L

    b. 100 L

    c. 350 L

    d. 1000 L

111. A return loop recycles water through the water treatment system because:

    a. it reduces the amount of water required.

    b. it prevents stagnant spots.

    c. of both a and b.

    d. of neither a nor b.

112. In a water treatment system, feed water is adjusted to a temperature of:

    a. 55oF, using a heater and cold water.

    b. 95oF, using a heater and cold water.

    c. 77°F–82°F, using hot water and a refrigeration unit.

    d. 77°F–82°F, using hot and cold water and a blending valve.

113. The pH of feed water is 9.0 at a certain center. Which of the following would be the best water treatment?

   a. No treatment is required
   b. Add hydrochloric acid to the feed water, using a mixing chamber
   c. Add sulfuric acid by direct injection into the water line
   d. Add sodium hydroxide to the feed water, using a mixing chamber

114. Which of the following statements about multimedia filters is correct?

   a. They trap successively smaller particles
   b. They trap successively larger particles
   c. They are backwashed with added solvent
   d. They are not necessary if an ultrafilter is present downstream

115. Water softeners remove calcium and magnesium by:

   a. ion exchange.
   b. adsorption.
   c. filtration.
   d. osmosis.

116. Which of the following statements about carbon tank removal of chlorine and chloramine from feed water is correct?

   a. It should use activated powdered charcoal
   b. It requires two carbon tanks in a series
   c. It may be done with a continuous flow of water
   d. It requires backwashing when the charcoal is exhausted

117. Which of the following statements about reverse osmosis is correct?

   a. There is a movement of water across a semipermeable membrane from a low-solute concentration to a high-solute concentration
   b. Prefiltration is not required
   c. Hydraulic pressure is used to move water through the membrane
   d. Solute concentration on both sides of the membrane becomes equal

118. Which of the following statements about the deionization of water is correct?

   a. It removes only cations
   b. It removes only anions
   c. It removes both anions and cations
   d. It uses on-site regenerated resins

119. Which of the following statements about an ultraviolet irradiator is correct?

   a. It emits light at a wavelength of 254 nanometers
   b. It has a glass sleeve through which water flows and that admits light
   c. It uses a hydrogen vapor lamp
   d. All of the above are true

120. Which of the following statements about biofilm is correct?

    a. It is easily removed from the water treatment system
    b. It does not adhere to surfaces
    c. It does not affect the water treatment system
    d. It is an aggregate of microorganisms that produce a matrix of extracellular polymeric substance (slime)

121. Public Law 92-603, which originally passed in 1972, is concerned with which of the following?

    a. It covers dialysis only
    b. It covers dialysis and kidney transplants
    c. It requires Medicare to pay 100% of dialysis treatments
    d. It set clinical requirements for dialysis patients

122. Which of the following statements best describes dialysis centers today?

    a. They are mostly owned by large dialysis organizations
    b. They are mostly hospital based
    c. They are overseen directly by Medicare
    d. None of the above describes dialysis centers

123. Inspection and standards for dialysis centers may be provided by:

    a. the Food and Drug Administration.
    b. state health departments.
    c. the Association for Advancement of Medical Instrumentation.
    d. all of the above.

124. Continuous quality improvement refers to:

    a. purifying water to make dialysate.
    b. improving the blood access surgery.
    c. a method for improving clinical, technical, and organizational procedures.
    d. a checklist of clinical data on a patient.

125. Professionalism for a hemodialysis technician includes:

    a. using a patient's first name or nickname to make the dialysis experience less formal.
    b. discussing personal problems with the patient as a way of sharing misfortune.
    c. keeping busy at all times to indicate that the technician is a critical member of the team.
    d. refraining from talking about a patient to a colleague if the conversation may be overheard.

126. Taking the Certified Clinical Hemodialysis Technician exam requires all of the following EXCEPT:

    a. 6-months of full-time (1000 hours) experience and training.
    b. a signature of a preceptor or supervisor to prove training and experience.
    c. compliance with state requirements for hemodialysis technicians.
    d. a high school diploma or GED.

127. Which of the following statements about certification examinations in clinical nephrology technology and in biomedical nephrology technology is correct?

a. They are given by different nephrology certification groups
b. They require 12 months of work experience to take the examination
c. They both require six major areas of knowledge in nephrology and dialysis
d. All of the above statements are correct

128. The National Kidney Foundation's Kidney Disease: Improving Global Outcomes includes treatment guidelines for all the following EXCEPT:

a. vascular access.
b. anemia.
c. hepatitis.
d. high blood pressure.

129. As part of the job of a dialysis technician, one may be required to lift equipment or assist with patient transfers. Back pain–sparing and injury prevention maneuvers include:

a. twisting the body to gain more power while lifting a heavy object.
b. pulling the heavy item; never pushing it.
c. lifting with the legs and holding the object close to the body.
d. trying to lift the object rapidly to avoid straining the back.

130. One difference between peritoneal dialysis (PD) and hemodialysis (HD) is:

a. there is a greater incidence of disequilibrium syndrome in PD.
b. there are more dietary restrictions in PD.
c. fluid buildup is less of a problem in HD.
d. the patient is subjected to constant dialysis in PD rather than intermittent dialysis in HD.

131. All of the following statements regarding kidney transplantation are correct EXCEPT:

a. the risk of death is in the 3%–5% range during the first year.
b. diabetes, heart disease, and older age decrease the success rate.
c. there is a 10%–15% lower success rate if the first transplant is rejected.
d. the diseased kidneys are usually removed.

132. Which of the following immunosuppressive drugs used in kidney transplant patients has renal toxicity?

a. Prednisone
b. Cyclosporine
c. Azathioprine
d. All of the above

133. What is a sensitization test for a potential kidney transplant recipient?

a. Human leukocyte antigen match
b. Blood group test
c. Potential recipient serum tested with a multiple donor lymphocyte panel
d. Potential donor serum tested with potential recipients' lymphocyte panel

134. A diet restricting all of the following is appropriate for a renal failure patient EXCEPT for:

    a. potassium.
    b. calcium.
    c. phosphate.
    d. fluids.

135. All of the following are indications to start hemodialysis in a renal failure patient EXCEPT:

    a. encephalopathy and seizures.
    b. serum potassium of 6.5 mEq/dL.
    c. serum creatinine of 15 mg/dL.
    d. creatinine clearance of 25 mL/min.

136. The nephrotic syndrome is characterized by all the following EXCEPT:

    a. hematuria.
    b. proteinuria greater than 3.5 g/d/1.72 m² body surface area.
    c. hyperlipidemia.
    d. hypoalbuminemia.

137. Which of the following statements about administering erythropoietin to a hemodialysis patient is correct?

    a. Administer it until the hemoglobin level is normal
    b. Give supplemental iron if ferritin is low
    c. Give it subcutaneously only
    d. Double the dose if the hemoglobin has not increased by 1 g/dL in 4 weeks

138. A recent study published in *The New England Journal of Medicine* compared hemodialysis three times a week with hemodialysis six times a week. At the end of a 12-month follow-up period, the study showed the six-times-a-week group had:

    a. a weekly Kt/V that was the same as in the three-times-a-week group.
    b. fewer deaths.
    c. the same left ventricular mass as in the three-times-a-week group.
    d. no difference with vascular access problems than in the three-times-a-week group

139. Which of the following statements about the nephron, the working unit of the kidney, is correct?

    a. It makes about 180 liters of glomerular filtrate a day
    b. Renal tubules deliver urine directly into the ureters
    c. Nephrons are found only in the renal cortex
    d. Bowman's capsule separates the collecting ducts from the renal tubules

140. Acute tubular necrosis may be caused by:

    a. shock and hypotension.
    b. rhabdomyolysis.
    c. radiographic contrast material.
    d. all of the above.

141. What does the expression _Kt/V_ signify with regard to hemodialysis?

    a. Blood flow through the dialyzer
    b. Dialysate flow through the dialyzer
    c. Prescribed dose of dialysis
    d. Formula for mixing water and concentrate

142. Adding extra sodium chloride to the dialysate will:

    a. draw water out of cells and tissues into the blood.
    b. decrease urine production during dialysis.
    c. reduce the amount of fluid that is ultrafiltered.
    d. have no effect on blood volume or fluid removal.

143. Which of the following is most likely to cause problems for the patient receiving hemodialysis treatments?

    a. Too lengthy dialysis session
    b. Inadequate vascular access
    c. Mistaken dialysis prescription
    d. Dietary indiscretion

144. Which of the following action is most important in preventing spread of infection?

    a. Wearing sterile gloves
    b. Autoclaving equipment
    c. Hand washing
    d. Wearing a sterile gown and mask

145. To avoid environmental contamination, it is important to do which of the following?

    a. Clean all surfaces at the station and the external portion of the dialysis machine
    b. Avoid storage of food and beverages in the same refrigerator or other container with blood or body fluid samples
    c. Place all used dialyzers and tubing in leak-proof containers
    d. Do all of the above

146. All of the following are part of a standard dialysis prescription EXCEPT:

    a. access to cannulate.
    b. length and frequency of treatment.
    c. dialysate composition.
    d. heparin dose.

147. A brother of a dialysis patient has blood type O and is being considered a potential kidney donor. What are the odds that he will be a complete match and a suitable donor?

    a. 25%
    b. 50%
    c. 75%
    d. 100%

148. A patient with kidney disease has anemia, fatigue, elevated phosphate levels, ankle edema, and elevated blood pressure. What is the most likely range of his glomerular filtration rate?

    a. 90–100 mL/min
    b. 60–90 mL/min
    c. 15–29 mL/min
    d. 5–15 mL/min

149. Which of the following physicians is credited with inventing dialysis?

    a. Willem J. Kolff, MD
    b. Belding H. Scribner, MD
    c. James A. Cimino, MD
    d. Gregory House, MD

150. What pattern of blood chemistries would you expect in renal osteodystrophy?

    a. High-calcium and low-phosphate levels
    b. Low–parathyroid hormone levels
    c. Elevated calcitriol
    d. Low-calcium and high-phosphate levels

Answer Key and Explanations

1. C: Hemodialysis requires vascular access since the blood flows out of the patient, through the dialysis machine's semipermeable membrane, and then back into the patient. The membrane keeps certain waste products or excess water from returning to the patient, while electrolytes and blood cells are returned. Peritoneal dialysis is performed with an intra-abdominal catheter without blood ever leaving the body. Vascular access is not required. The blood vessels of the abdominal cavity act as a filter similar to the semipermeable membrane used in hemodialysis. Peritoneal dialysis may be performed at home with a cycler machine to exchange fresh sterile dialysate, often overnight 7 days a week. Manual exchange of dialysate may also be done.

2. B: Since hemodialysis must be carried out repetitively, usually three times a week for 4 hours, repeated vascular access is required. Arterial blood is sent to the dialyzer and returned to the patient by an arm vein. Arteriovenous shunts connect the artery and vein by an external tube, which has a connecting port so that blood may be sent to the dialysis machine from the artery and returned to the vein. These shunts are subject to infection and clotting so that surgically implanted arteriovenous fistulas were developed, which connect artery and vein entirely within the arm. These are still standard for most dialysis patients.

3. D: Dialysis machines have evolved since their initial frequent use in the 1960s. The initial type, the so-called Kiil, consisted of 70 lb. flat plates covered by sheets of cellophane. They required cleaning and storage after each use, and membranes had to be replaced. The coil dialyzer was supported by a mesh screen coiled around a central core. It required complete sterilization with a large amount of blood in a canister that was bathed in the dialysate. The Gambro flat plate dialyzer used a new membrane type named cuprophane. These early machines were replaced by the so-called hollow fiber dialyzer, which is the type in use today. In this model, the blood flows through tiny hollow tubes (fibers) while the dialysate flows around the outside of these fibers. Biocompatible membranes, sophisticated alarms, and automatic functions characterize the modern dialyzer.

4. A: The kidney is a fist-sized bilateral organ with a tough outer capsule. The most external portion of the organ is called the cortex. The renal medulla or interior portion of the kidney contains sections called pyramids with points referred to as papillae. Each papilla delivers urine into a receptacle-like calyx, which then transmits urine into the renal pelvis. The pelvis connects to the ureter and delivers urine for excretion. The functional unit of the kidney is the nephron, present in the cortex and extending into the medulla. The nephron is composed of a glomerulus, a tangled bunch of capillaries, which produces the glomerular filtrate, and a renal tubule, which acts on the filtrate to reabsorb water and exchange electrolytes. Blood is conducted to the glomerulus via an afferent arteriole and is filtered by the glomerular capillaries, which retain blood cells and large molecules, such as proteins. The blood is then returned by way of an efferent arteriole.

5. C: The normal adult has a glomerular filtration rate (GFR) of about 125 mL/min, although there is some variability due to age and sex. Clinically, this value is often expressed as GFR/m^2 body surface area. It is usually measured by the so-called creatinine clearance in which blood and urine creatinine concentrations and the urine volume are measured, and the GFR calculated. Little creatinine is reabsorbed by the renal tubules, thus making it a valuable standard for estimating glomerular function. In end stage renal disease, the GFR is often below 15 mL/min/1.73 m^2, and dialysis is required. Many drugs are excreted by the kidneys, and dosage adjustments based on GFR are often necessary.

6. B: In addition to its role in water and electrolyte balance and acid–base control, the kidney also produces substances that are of importance in erythropoiesis, vitamin D metabolism, and blood pressure control. Production of the hormone erythropoietin by juxtaglomerular renal cells is important in controlling red blood cell production in the bone marrow. In the presence of anemia, the resulting hypoxia stimulates the hypoxia-inducible transcription factor in these cells, and increased amounts of erythropoietin are produced. A decrease in renal perfusion leads to increased production of renin by the kidney; this enzyme catalyzes the conversion of angiotensinogen to angiotensin 1, which is subsequently converted to angiotensin 2 by an angiotensin-converting enzyme. The latter stimulates aldosterone secretion by the adrenal gland. The renin–angiotensin–aldosterone system is of great importance in the regulation of blood pressure. The active form of vitamin D, calcitriol, is also produced in the kidney.

7. D: Acute renal failure (ARF) is usually classified by the anatomic location of the damage. Pre–renal failure typically is caused by hypotension, resulting from trauma, dehydration, or blood loss in which the renal blood flow is markedly diminished. Intrarenal failure is caused by intrinsic kidney diseases, such as glomerulonephritis or renal toxic drugs, such as certain antibiotics, chemotherapy agents, or radiologic contrast materials. Post–renal failure may be caused by problems distal to the kidney that cause obstruction to urine flow, such as ureteral calculi, kinked ureter, neoplastic invasion, or prostatic hypertrophy in men. ARF may proceed to chronic renal failure but may resolve with careful medical treatment and sometimes hemodialysis.

8. A: Diabetes mellitus is the commonest cause of chronic renal failure (CRF) in the United States. Because of the obesity epidemic, type 2 diabetes (90% of diabetic patients) is on the rise, and thus, there may be even more cases of CRF in the future. Diabetic nephropathy is most likely caused by endovascular damage to the renal vessels. Hypertension is the second leading cause of CRF. It is most often of the so-called essential type in which the exact cause is unknown. In the first few years of this decade, about 27% of patients on dialysis had kidney failure as a result of hypertension. Renal disease or renal artery stenosis may also cause hypertension with its deleterious effects. Additional causes of CRF include glomerular diseases and polycystic disease. Less common causes of CRF are cancer, kidney infections, AIDS, systemic lupus erythematosus, and sickle cell disease.

9. D: Uremia is the term given to a constellation of symptoms resulting from kidney failure, with a resultant buildup of waste products in the circulation (e.g., urea), Some of the typical symptoms include fatigue (often resulting from anemia, which is common in chronic renal disease), itching, myalgias, dyspnea or edema from fluid retention, skin pallor or yellowish cast, foamy urine (due to protein), and nocturia. Loss of protein in the urine greater than 3.5 g/d is referred to as the nephrotic syndrome and may be a cause of excessive fluid retention. Often these symptoms develop gradually so frequent inquiry of the patient is indicated. Hemodialysis may improve uremic symptoms, but it only reproduces about 15% of normal kidney function; thus, an increased frequency and duration of hemodialysis may be indicated if the symptoms persist. Urinary tract infections are caused by the introduction of bacteria, not by uremia.

10. B: Numerous abnormalities of the blood, protein, and electrolytes occur in chronic renal failure. Anemia is very common due to frequent blood loss with resulting iron deficiency and diminished secretion of erythropoietin by the diseased kidney. Calcium absorption is impaired due to inadequate calcitriol, and phosphate is not adequately excreted by the tubules, resulting in elevated phosphate levels. A low calcium level stimulates the parathyroid gland to produce more parathyroid hormone, producing so-called secondary hyperparathyroidism. This may result in calcium deposition in the heart and blood vessels. Elevated potassium levels are also quite common in these patients and may be life-threatening.

11. A: Kidney transplant has become a major form of treatment for chronic renal disease. About 15,000 are done each year in the United States. The donor kidney may be from a living related individual (e.g., brother or sister), a living non-related donor (e.g., spouse or friend), or a cadaver kidney, usually from a non-related individual who has died recently. In the latter case, the patient is usually matched from the national donor list. Living donors should be in good physical and mental health, and in all cases, blood and tissue type (human leukocyte antigen) matching is very important for the survival of the organ in the recipient. The transplanted kidney may last up to 20 years or more, nearly always with the use of immunosuppressant drugs that lower the chance of rejection. About 89%–95% of transplanted kidneys are functional at 1-year post-surgery.

12. C: Most hemodialysis in the United States is done in centers, usually 3–4 hours a session, 3 days a week. The presence of nurses, technicians, and other patients is often reassuring to the individual undergoing treatment. However, the time commitment may interfere with work schedules or parenting of young children. Some centers offer night treatment with the patient sleeping over while having hemodialysis. Home hemodialysis, using dialyzers appropriately designed for home use, is another option, but the patient and spouse or partner must undergo training regarding techniques and standard procedures and a plan of action in emergencies. Nocturnal home hemodialysis during sleep allows prolonged treatment and has been shown to reduce many of the symptoms of chronic renal disease. Probably the most efficient schedule is that of the newer short daily home hemodialysis, usually 2–3 hours a session, 5–7 days a week. The initial 2 hours of dialysis are the most efficient, and the shortened time schedule allows more time for work and recreational activities.

13. C: Since there is little or no urine production in patients with end-stage renal disease, excess fluid must be removed by dialysis. The volume of urine that the patient does produce plus so-called insensible losses (e.g., breathing, stool, perspiration), around 600 mL/d, is the usual fluid replacement formula. Thus, a typical prescription would be urine volume plus 1 L (4 cups) a day. Close attention to dry weight (post-dialysis weight) and symptoms of dehydration (e.g., thirst, weight loss, poor skin turgor, hypotension) or fluid overload (e.g., edema, pulmonary congestion, hypertension) must be a part of the evaluation of every patient. Since loss of appetite and malnutrition are common in these patients, dietary considerations are very important, and consultation with a dietitian trained in renal failure is often necessary.

14. B: Beta$_2$-microglobulin is a protein widely distributed on cell surfaces and in body fluids. It is a precursor of the protein amyloid, which is formed when the beta$_2$-microglobulin enters tissues and is converted to amyloid. Healthy kidneys remove excess beta$_2$-microglobulin, but in renal failure, levels rise, and so-called amyloidosis occurs. This may lead to carpal tunnel syndrome, joint pain, bone cysts, compression fractures, and cutaneous bleeding. Nearly 20% of hemodialysis patients develop amyloidosis after 10 years and 80%–100% after 29 years. Pericarditis, inflammation, and fluid accumulation within the pericardium, is common in chronic renal disease as is peripheral neuropathy, most likely due to inadequate excretion of neurotoxic substances. Seizures may occur but are usually related to electrolyte abnormalities, especially hyponatremia.

15. A: Ferritin is the main storage protein for iron, required for hemoglobin synthesis, and is usually low in iron deficiency anemia. Most patients with chronic renal failure are anemic, usually from inadequate erythropoietin production by the kidney or bleeding, often gastrointestinal, or both. Erythropoietin levels may be checked, but drugs, such as Epogen or Procrit, that stimulate red cell production will not work effectively unless iron stores are adequate. The use of these erythropoiesis-stimulatory agents is quite common in hemodialysis patients, aiming for a hemoglobin level in the 10–12 g/dL range. Blood transfusions may thus be avoided. Iron supplementation may be required to keep the ferritin level above 200 ng/mL. It should be checked monthly. A potential source of blood loss should be investigated.

16. D: Hyperphosphatemia (elevated serum phosphate) is common in chronic renal failure patients since the kidneys are unable to excrete this substance. Low calcium and elevated phosphate levels are typical of these patients and lead to secondary hyperparathyroidism and bone loss (renal osteodystrophy). A low phosphate diet, calcium supplements with vitamin D, and phosphate binders are all useful in limiting high phosphate levels. High phosphate foods include chocolate, dairy products, dried beans, nuts, pizza, and cola drinks. Calcium supplements with vitamin D may also be useful in controlling the elevated phosphate. The most effective agents are phosphate binders, which bind to phosphate in the gastrointestinal tract and prevent absorption. Of these, the nonaluminum and calcium-containing compounds (e.g., lanthanum carbonate) are preferred because there is less toxicity.

17. D: Engaging the patient in his or her own care usually has positive benefits. This is especially true for patients who wish to do home dialysis. The technical staff should assess the patient's capacity for these techniques and their implications. The more skillful the patient is with needle placement to the access site, choosing the right foods, calculating weight and fluid status, and checking the dialyzer and dialysate, the more likely he or she will have a positive attitude toward the treatment and prognosis. The same is true for a spouse or other caregiver. Learning for what each medication is needed and watching out for specific symptoms are also important for patient education and safety.

18. A: Dialysis does remove some water-soluble vitamins, such as biotin, folate, niacin, pantothenic acid (vitamin B_5), thiamine, and riboflavin so supplements of these are recommended. Patients should take 60–100 mg of vitamin C and 800–1000 mcg folic acid daily. Exact doses in multivitamin tablets should be checked. Megadose vitamin therapy is not recommended. The healthy kidney may excrete high vitamin doses, but toxic levels may accumulate as dialysis is unlikely to handle large doses. This is especially true of fat-soluble vitamins A and D and possibly E and K. Over-the-counter herbs and food supplements should be discussed with a medical professional before using them.

19. B: Diffusion refers to the movement of solute through a semipermeable membrane from a high concentration to a low concentration, a so-called concentration gradient. Unlike hydrostatic pressure, no external force is required; the molecules supply their own energy. In time the solute concentration on both sides of the membrane equalizes. Factors that influence the speed of diffusion include the size and number of the membrane pores, the size of the solute molecules (molecular weight), and the temperature of the solution. Osmosis refers to the movement of solvent through the semipermeable membrane from a low-solute concentration to a high-solute concentration, sometimes referred to as movement of solvent from low-osmotic pressure or osmolality to high-osmotic pressure or osmolality. Both processes occur across living cell membranes and in dialysis.

20. B: In hemodialysis, both diffusion and osmosis occur. The dialysate is prepared with solutes (e.g., ions, glucose) to achieve desired levels in the blood. More efficient exchange of fluid and solute is obtained if the two fluids flow in opposite directions, a so-called countercurrent exchange. This is because the gradients can be maintained for the entire length of the tubing, speeding up the elimination of waste products (e.g., urea). Flow of both fluids in the same direction would decrease the diffusion and osmotic gradients over the length of the fiber and would be less efficient. Excess water may be removed, using hydraulic pressure and ultrafiltration through a filter that traps large molecules (e.g., proteins) and blood cells. So-called convective transport may occur, leading to solvent drag in which solvent crossing the semipermeable membrane drags along smaller solutes.

21. B: Body fluids are present in three different sites, known as compartments. The fluid inside cells is referred to as the intracellular compartment. The fluid between cells is called the interstitial compartment. Blood in vessels makes up the intravascular compartment. Differences in osmotically active solute concentration (gradients) in different compartments cause water to flow toward a state of equilibrium. Hemodialysis acts only on blood that is removed from the access site (intravascular blood), pumped through the hollow fibers of the dialyzer, which has a semipermeable membrane that separates the blood from the dialysate, and is then returned to the body. Water flows through the membrane to the higher osmotically active fluid, largely determined by the sodium concentration and with some contribution from other osmotically active molecules.

22. B: In hemodialysis, arterial blood is conducted through tubing to a pump, which forces the blood through the hollow fibers in the dialyzer. The pre-pump blood usually has a negative pressure, while the post-pump blood (arterial header) about to enter the hollow fibers has the highest positive pressure, the value depending on the resistance of the fibers. Pressure then diminishes over the length of the fiber, and the pressure in the venous return is the lowest positive pressure in the system. The dialysis machine can control the pressure differential between the dialysate and the blood, the so-called transmembrane pressure. This may be adjusted to control the amount of fluid removal. The average pressure difference between blood entering and leaving the dialyzer fibers determines the net hydraulic pressure, forcing fluid out of the blood, through the membrane, and into the dialysate.

23. A: As water moves through the membrane from the blood to the dialysate (convection), it drags molecules along with it (solvent drag). The size of the molecule and the size and number of the pores in the membrane determine the fraction of solute that undergoes convective transport. Small molecules pass easily and quickly, but large molecules pass more slowly. The term "sieving coefficient of a membrane" refers to the amount of a given solute that passes through the membrane from the blood into the dialysate. A sieving coefficient of 1.0 indicates that 100% of a given solute passed through the membrane, while a sieving coefficient of 0.4 indicates that only 40% of a given solute passed through the membrane by a convective mechanism.

24. C: Osmotic forces determine which way water will move from one body fluid compartment to another. In hemodialysis, water is forced through the membrane by ultrafiltration so that the solute concentration of the blood is lowered. Water is then returned to the cells and tissues from the blood by osmotic forces since the cellular osmotically active solute concentration is now higher than in the blood. This may result in a fall in blood volume and result in hypotension. Sodium may be added to the dialysate, which will then increase the osmolality of the blood, pulling water out of the cells and tissues. The sodium in the dialysate is then lowered later in the dialysis process so that the excess water can be removed from the blood. Ultrafiltration occurs within the dialyzer but not within the body compartments. Active transport may drive ion exchange across cellular membranes, but water movement is passive and determined by osmotic forces.

25. D: Biocompatibility refers to the interaction of the membrane with the blood contents. Touching of blood to the membrane may activate certain cellular or protein elements in the blood, causing immunologic reactions, such as allergic reactions or anaphylaxis. Release of deleterious cytokines or enhanced clotting may occur. Adsorption of blood proteins onto the fiber wall tends to improve biocompatibility since the material is no longer seen as "foreign" by immunocompetent cells. In general, synthetic membranes are more biocompatible than those of cellulose due to their ability to absorb proteins better than the latter. Reprocessed (cleaned and reused) dialyzers may be more biocompatible than new ones since they retain some adsorbed protein (unless bleach is used to strip off the protein).

26. C: For ultrafiltration to force fluid through the semipermeable membrane, the hydraulic pressure in the blood compartment must be higher than in the dialysate compartment. This pressure difference is referred to as a hydraulic pressure gradient or a transmembrane pressure. The pressures in each compartment may be set by the dialysis machine. A simple method of calculating the amount of fluid to be removed is by subtracting the estimated dry weight (EDW) of the patient from his or her pre-dialysis weight (PRW). Any fluid given during the procedure may then be added to the difference. Assuming 1 L of water weighs 1 kg, the EDW is 75 kg, the PRW is 80 kg, and the patient receives 0.5 L during the treatment. Thus, the amount of fluid to be removed would be: 80 – 75 + 0.5 = 5.5 L.

27. A: The dialysis machine can alter the hydraulic pressures in the blood and dialysate compartments and thus control the ultrafiltration rate of the fluid transfer. Each dialyzer has an ultrafiltration coefficient (Kuf) determined by the manufacturer. This refers to the volume of fluid (in mL) that passes through the membrane at a given pressure difference in 1 hour. Thus, a dialyzer with a Kuf of 5 and a transmembrane pressure of 50 mm Hg transfers 250 mL (5 x 50) of fluid in 1 hour of dialysis. Patients with kidney failure are often edematous with excess water in the interstitial compartment so that removal by dialysis represents an efficient way of controlling fluid volume and weight. Since the patient's kidneys are not functioning, diuretic drugs are of little benefit.

28. C: Molecular weights of a chemical compound represent the sum of the atomic weights of the atoms that make up the molecule. Each dialyzer membrane has a molecular weight cutoff (in daltons) that determines the size of the molecules that can pass through it. These may range from 3000 to 15,000 daltons. Small molecules (e.g., sodium, potassium, phosphate, urea, water) pass through the filter easily, while large molecules, such as proteins (e.g., albumin with a molecular weight of 66,000 daltons) cannot. Choosing the appropriate molecular cutoff for a membrane helps to determine what size molecule may be removed from the blood. This is particularly important for drug overdoses and toxins.

29. B: The volume of blood that can be cleared of a given solute per unit time is referred to as clearance (K). The clearance for a given solute is given by the manufacturer based on blood and dialysis flow rates; membrane characteristics; and the molecular weight, size, and charge of the solute. Most low-molecular weight solutes are removed during dialysis by diffusion from the high-concentration to the low-concentration side of the membrane with the rate also dependent on temperature. Large molecules tend to cross the membrane by convection (solvent drag). The sieving coefficient (SC) indicates the amount of solute passing through the membrane with the rest rejected or adsorbed. Thus, an SC of 0.4 predicts that 40% of a given solute will pass through the membrane. Mostly small proteins are removed from the blood by adsorption to the membrane, although cellulose membranes tend to absorb more than synthetic hydrophobic ones. Membranes with adsorbed material are more biocompatible but may diminish diffusion and convection.

30. A: A hollow fiber dialyzer holds thousands of fiber tubes through which the blood flows. They are surrounded by dialysate, separated by the membrane. The blood and dialysate flow in opposite directions, a so-called countercurrent mechanism, which enhances molecular exchange. This is because the concentration gradients are little changed from one end of the fiber to the other. The hollow fibers are very thin but rigid so that the membrane compliance (deformability or volume change) is low. Ultrafiltration rates are predictable so that precise amounts of fluid removal may be accomplished. The hollow filters have a low resistance to blood flow so that there is not much volume difference at low and high pressure.

31. B: Dialysis membranes may be of three types: cellulose, modified cellulose, and synthetic. Cellulose membranes have thin fiber walls, and solutes pass through them mostly by diffusion. The molecular cutoff is low, about 3000 daltons, so that intermediate-size molecular passage (e.g., beta$_2$-microglobulin at 11,800 daltons) is limited. They are also the least biocompatible of the three types since adsorption is limited. Modified-cellulose membranes have the hydroxyl groups of the molecule replaced by acetate, amino acids, or other synthetic molecules. Their adsorption is improved, and diffusion, convection, and adsorption of solute are better than cellulose. The most effective membranes are purely synthetic made of polymers (e.g., polysulfone, polymethacrylate) formed into hollow fibers with thick walls. These membranes can remove solute up to 15,000 daltons in size, and their adsorption is quite good, leading to an improved biocompatibility.

32. B: A dialyzer's clearance rate for a particular solute indicates the volume of blood from which the solute will be removed per unit time. It is usually expressed as a K value in mL/min. Thus, with a K of 200 mL/min for urea, 200 mL of the 300 mL blood flowing through in 1 minute will be cleared of urea in 1 minute. Of course, blood is continually recirculated through the dialyzer so a considerable amount of urea may be removed. Blood flow rate (Qb) may be increased to lessen the time of dialysis, but there is a rate limit due to the amount of blood that can flow through the needle in the patient's vascular access. Dialysis flow rate (Qd) may also increase clearance but to a lesser degree.

33. D: The manufacturer's stated clearance for a particular solute is based on laboratory analysis of watery fluids that only approximate the rheological properties of blood. The actual value may differ by ± 10%–30%. Urea is the solute most frequently employed. The true clearance may be calculated by measuring the concentration of the solute going in and coming out of the dialyzer. The formula for dialyzer solute clearance is: $K = (Cb_i – Cb_o)/Cb_i \times Qb$, where K is the clearance, Cb_i is the inlet solute concentration (arterial), Cb_o is the outlet solute concentration (venous), and Qb is the blood flow in mL/min. Increasing the dialysate flow rate (Qd) may slightly improve the solute clearance, but this is not a part of the formula.

34. D: The dialysate composition contains ions and glucose in concentrations similar to those of the blood. Usually two concentrates are prepared: acid (contains sodium, potassium, magnesium, calcium, chloride, and glucose) and bicarbonate buffer. Acetic acid is added to the acid solution to adjust the pH. The two concentrates are then mixed and diluted with treated water. The concentrates come in three different formulations so it is important to mix the compatible ones. The final concentrations of the ions are adjusted, depending on whether one wishes to raise or lower their blood concentration. Thus, for a hyperkalemic (high potassium) patient, one might not add any potassium or keep it lower than the blood concentration. Phosphate is not routinely added to the dialysate.

35. A: Usually sodium concentration in the dialysate is kept the same or similar to that of the blood: 135–145 mEq/L. However, higher concentrates are sometimes used at the outset to drive sodium into the blood and raise its concentration. This then enhances an osmotic fluid shift from the interstitial space into the blood and accelerates fluid withdrawal. Then the sodium concentration is slowly reduced during the course of the dialysis, a process called sodium modeling. Caution must be used when performing this procedure since increased thirst and hypertension may result. The physician usually prescribes the concentration of sodium and the speed with which it is reduced.

36. A: Conductivity refers to an electrical method of measuring the electrolytes in the dialysate. Most dialysis units have two conductivity meters, one for the initial concentrate mixture and one for the final dialysate. Electrodes or sensor cells may be employed to measure the current generated by the ionic strength of the solution. The conductivity is monitored in a so-called redundant fashion so that two monitors are used to protect patient safety. Alarms and automatic bypass systems warn of errors in the dialysate composition, and the fluid is diverted to a drain before reaching the patient. Low conductivity is the most common cause of alarm, usually due to low-concentrate levels. A high-conductivity alarm may indicate poor water flow to the proportioning system, untreated incoming water, or use of the wrong dialysate concentrate.

37. B: Dialysate is made by mixing treated fresh water with concentrates containing the appropriate salts and glucose. The exact amounts of water and concentrate to be mixed depend on the dialysis center and the needs of a particular patient. There must be adequate volumes of water and concentrate for the entire procedure. Mixing of concentrate and water may be accomplished by two different methods: (1) by fixed-ratio pumps in which a diaphragm or piston pump delivers water and concentrate, according to a preset formula; or (2) by a servo-controlled mechanism in which the proportions of water and concentrate are automatically adjusted based on the conductance of the mixture, which is set to a prescribed level.

38. B: High-flux dialysis is a new, more efficient method of hemodialysis than the conventional method. The dialyzer has larger pores for more rapid removal of uremic toxins. Because of the large pores in the membrane, this method can remove larger molecules than the traditional method, for example $beta_2$-microglobulin, which is thought to contribute to arthritis in uremic patients and predisposes to amyloid deposition. The dialysis procedure can also be speeded up by increasing the blood flow to 450 mL/min, which is not possible in the traditional method. Speeding up the rate of flow of the dialysate is also possible. The unit contains an ultrafiltration controller device to regulate the volume of fluid removed from the patient from very small amounts up to 4 L/hr.

39. C: Bicarbonate buffer is used for the dialysate since the acetate previously used caused vasodilation and hypotension. Immunologic reactions and fluctuations in the white blood cell count are less common since the membranes used are more biocompatible. Pyrogenic reactions in high-flux dialysis are common, causing fever and discomfort for the patient, and sometimes require hospitalization for observation. This may be because the high-flux membranes have larger pores that allow fragments of bacterial particles to pass into the blood. Such pyrogens have been found in the dialysate. Generally, patients experience less post-dialysis fatigue and may in fact feel better because of the more efficient removal and shorter dialysis times.

40. D: Some patients may choose to have dialysis at home rather than adhere to a fixed schedule at a center. This is often true of people still employed, although some centers do night dialysis. In general, a spouse or other family member must be available to assist the patient. Both patient and assistant must undergo training for 6–8 weeks. Some vendors that supply home-dialysis equipment may also supply a visiting dialysis nurse if no home-based assistant is available. Most centers do not have night schedules, and food is not permitted during the procedure. At home, the end stage renal disease patient may snack during dialysis and even undergo the procedure during sleep, if there is an assistant who remains awake. The flexibility of home dialysis appeals to many patients, but some patients feel more secure at a dialysis center.

41. A: Dialysate is controlled in an optimum temperature range, usually between 38°C–40°C. Temperatures above 41°C may cause red blood cell hemolysis. Lower temperatures are usually not dangerous but may be uncomfortable for the patient who may complain of feeling cold. Lower temperatures generally diminish diffusion and thus increase dialysis time. Temperatures are usually controlled by a thermistor-controlled heater, although some systems use a heat exchanger to transfer heat from used dialysate to incoming cold water, thus saving energy. A separate temperature monitor is present before the dialysate enters the dialyzer and is equipped with preset temperature limits and alarms to signal departure from these limits. Incoming water must be warmed to a certain temperature before mixing with concentrate.

42. D: Dialysate flow is controlled by a pump. This pump may be preset by the manufacturer to deliver a fixed flow rate but usually can be varied, according to prescription in most systems. High-flow rates improve efficiency of dialysis and may deliver dialysate at rates from 0–1000 mL/min. Little improvement is noted with rates over 800 mL/min. There are visual and audible alarms for several different interruptions or abnormalities in the dialysate flow, such as low water pressure, pump failure, obstruction to flow, or power failure. Conductivity, pH, and temperature outside a preset range may set off alarms or blood leaks in some systems.

43. B: Blood leaks through a defect in the dialyzer membrane occur and represent a source of potential trouble. The leak may be large and cause significant blood loss and resulting hypotension. The blood may also be exposed to nonsterile dialysate, and there is a risk of contamination; thus, it should not be returned to the patient. Blood is detected in the dialysate by a light source and photocell or photoresistor, which is often sensitive enough to detect very small amounts of blood. In some units, the sensitivity may be adjusted. A blood leak will trigger an alarm and stop the flow of blood by signaling the blood pump and clamping the venous line. The volume of blood leakage may be grossly detected by inspecting the dialysate and testing it with a blood detecting strip (e.g., Hemastix). If blood is seen, the leak is large; clear dialysate with a positive strip test suggests a small leak; clear dialysate with a negative strip test suggests a false alarm.

44. A: The pH value indicates how acidic or basic a solution is with 7.0 considered neutral; that is, there are an equal number of acidic and basic ions. Values below 7.0 indicate an acidic solution, and values above 7.0 indicate a basic solution. Buffer solutions (e.g., bicarbonate) are used to maintain the pH at or near a certain level. Normal blood pH is in the 7.35–7.45 range. This may be affected by the dialysate so the pH of the latter is usually kept in the 7.0–7.4 range. In most dialysis systems, the pH of the dialysate is monitored continuously. Even if the system is so equipped, the initial pH of the dialysate should be checked by manual means. This is usually by a pH-sensitive dipstick with a color code to indicate the pH value.

45. B: Excess fluid in the blood may be removed into the dialysate, depending on the relative pressures on either side of the membrane, the so-called transmembrane pressure (TMP). Obviously, the blood pressure needs to be higher than the dialysate pressure to form a gradient to direct the direction of water flow. In older machines, a technician was required to determine the amount of fluid to be removed from the patient and calculate the hourly ultrafiltration rate (UFR). Mathematical formulae were then used to find the TMP needed for the ultrafiltration constant (Kuf) of a particular dialyzer. Newer machines have their own systems to control UFR by either volume or flow modification of the dialysate. The fluid volume (in mL) to be removed and the treatment time are entered, and the machine sets the TMP. The Kuf reported by the dialyzer manufacturer is based on in-vitro determination and is usually higher than the actual in-vivo value.

46. C: Dialysis systems are able to control the amount of fluid removed from the patient per unit time. This amount is controlled by either volume or flow regulation. The former uses a volumetric balancing system by use of two equal volume chambers, each separated by a flexible diaphragm. Used dialysate enters one chamber, displaces the diaphragm to force an equal volume of fresh dialysate to the dialyzer. The used dialysate is then sent to the drain. A flow pump sets the rate at which fresh dialyzer enters one chamber and another drives used dialysate to the other chamber. A second, less common method is by flow control in which sensors monitor the flow rate of dialysate to and from the dialyzer. The flow is balanced on either side of the dialyzer by inlet and outlet pumps. Both types of control mechanisms are computer driven.

165

47. D: The extracorporeal circuit refers to the system of tubes, drip chambers, pressure gauges, and pump that connect the arterial and venous accesses to the dialyzer. The drip chambers have gauges to measure arterial and venous pressures by monitoring lines with transducer protectors. The drip chamber also traps any air that gets into the line and prevents blood clots in the extracorporeal circulation from entering the patient by use of a fine wire mesh on the venous side before the patient's venous access. The arterial blood is propelled from the drip chamber into the dialyzer by a blood pump in which the pliable and slightly larger-in-diameter arterial tubing is threaded through the pump rollers.

48. A: The amount of patient's blood in the extracorporeal system is controlled in the dialysis procedure, usually in the 100–250 mL range, so that hypovolemic hypotension does not occur. The arterial access needle has a relatively small bore and is the rate-limiting segment. Blood lines are smooth and narrow to reduce clotting and air bubbles; the arterial tubing is usually colored red, and the venous tubing, blue. The tubing may be custom-made to be compatible with certain dialysis units and patient requirements. Anticoagulation with heparin is usually given through a small diameter tube that connects to the arterial blood tubing. Saline infusions are possible through an accessory line just before the arterial blood pump.

49. D: A transducer in the dialysis pathway is a pressure-sensitive device that converts pressure into an electronic signal. This signal displays venous, arterial, and transmembrane pressures. They connect to arterial and venous ports in the arterial input and venous output lines by a small tube at the top of the drip chambers. Transducer protectors are connected to the end of these lines. They use membranes of 0.2 micron that are hydrophobic to keep fluid from passing through. Wet or clamped transducer protectors cause pressure reading errors, and damaged ones may admit air on the arterial side. The Centers for Disease Control safety alert recommend changing wet transducer protectors to prevent cross contamination. It may be necessary to change the machine's internal transducer protector (a backup) and disinfect the system before the next dialysis treatment.

50. D: Blood flow into the dialyzer is accomplished with a blood pump, usually a roller type, which compresses the blood tubing and promotes forward motion of the blood. The volume of blood entering the dialyzer may, thus, be controlled by the speed of the rotating roller, which may be set by the technician. Typical blood flow volumes range from 0–600 mL/min. The flow rate may be specified by the physician's prescription. A high negative pressure flattens the tubing in the roller pump and diminishes the volume of blood delivered so that the indicated flow by the roller pump may be greater than the volume actually delivered. A manual cranking system is available on most pumps in case of emergency and may be used to keep the venous pressure below the alarm level.

51. A: While arterial pressure in the patient is positive (e.g., mean pressure of 100 mm Hg), the pressure from the patient's arterial access, also called the pre-pump pressure, is usually negative. This is because the source is from a fistula or graft, and resistance from the vascular access and the pulling of the pump creates a negative pressure. The pre-dialyzer or post-dialyzer pump pressure is that of the blood between the pump and the dialyzer and is positive, the highest in the system. The post-dialyzer or venous pressure is positive, but lower than the pre-dialyzer pressure. A large pressure differential on either side of the dialyzer suggests a clot in the system and will set off an alarm in most dialysis systems.

52. C: The pre-pump pressure monitor will set off an alarm if the pressure is above or below the preset limits. Several mishaps or therapeutic maneuvers may set off the high-pressure alarm: a bloodline separation (if the upper limit is set below zero), a leak between the patient and the monitoring site, a decrease in the blood pump speed, and infusion of saline or medications. A low-pressure alarm may sound if there is blockage of arterial flow from the arterial needle, compression of the arterial tubing, hypotension, or a pump rate higher than the vascular access can supply. Vasoconstriction of the patient's vessels or a poorly working central catheter may also set off a low-pressure alarm.

53. D: Post-dialyzer or venous pressure is that in the tubing returning blood from the dialyzer to the patient's venous access. A low-pressure alarm may be set off by a separation of the blood tubing from the venous needle or catheter, a fall in the blood flow rate, a blockage in the tubing before the venous monitor, or a major clot in the dialyzer. The high-pressure venous alarm may be set off by a blockage of the blood tubing between the monitoring site and the patient's venous access, poor positioning or infiltration of the venous needle, a poorly working central venous catheter, or a clot in the venous access.

54. B: Air that enters the patient's circulation (air embolism) is potentially lethal and must be prevented. Dialyzer systems are equipped with air detectors that monitor the post-dialyzer venous line. These function by an ultrasonic mechanism (sound travels faster through air than liquid) or a photocell apparatus that measures the difference in light transmission between air and liquid. The monitor sets off an alarm if air is detected, and a venous line clamp is activated to shut off the blood flow to the venous access. The blood pump may also be stopped automatically. The sensitivity of the alarm is usually preset by the manufacturer but may be adjusted by a qualified technician. The technician must always be certain the air detector is functional and that the venous blood clamp is present and functional.

55. D: To prevent blood in the dialysis system from clotting, the anticoagulant heparin is given into the post-pump (pre-dialyzer) tubing. This may be done by a full dose bolus or intermittent injection at set times during the procedure. Heparin infusion, using a syringe and a rate-controlling motor to drive the syringe plunger at a preset rate through a heparin infusion line, is most often used. Most heparin lines are connected after the blood pump so that the pre-pump negative pressure does not draw air into the system by way of the heparin line. Heparin is usually stopped before the end of treatment so that the blood returns to its normal coagulability by the end of the dialysis session. It is critical that the correct heparin dose be given to avoid excessive bleeding.

56. C: A sorbent is material that has the capacity to absorb liquids or gases. It may function as a molecular sieve because it has a large internal surface area and is typically composed of pellets 1–2 mm in diameter and up to 5 mm in length. Some sorbents have a high affinity for absorbing other substances. In a sorbent dialysis cartridge, there are several layers, such as zirconium oxide and zirconium carbonate and activated charcoal, which absorb chemicals from the used dialysate and regenerate fresh dialysate. The sorbent cartridge also serves as a continuous disinfection system for the dialysate by removing bacteria and endotoxins. The patient's ultrafiltrate is also converted into dialysate by passage through the sorbent cartridge.

57. B: A sorbent dialysis system does not require a continuous source of treated water. A chemical mixture is added to 6 liters of tap water, which is purified by cycling the resulting dialysate through a cartridge with several sorbents. The usual cartridge has four layers. It removes calcium, potassium, and magnesium from the used dialysate since the concentrations of these chemicals were altered by passage through the dialyzer. These chemicals are then added back into the fresh dialysate by an infusion system. Different cartridges are available, and depending on which one is used, the time of dialysis may be short (3–5 hours) at dialysis flow rates of 400 mL/min or slow (5–8 hours) at rates of 200–3000 mL/min.

58. B: An arteriovenous fistula is surgically created by connecting an artery to a vein (anastamosis), usually in the forearm. Other sites may be used if there is damage or previous surgery on the vessels at this site. The vein undergoes arterialization because of the high arterial pressure and becomes thicker and more accessible to needle penetration. There are four surgical methods of connecting artery to vein: (1) arterial side to venous side, which provides good blood flow, is the easiest to perform by the surgeon, but may result in swelling of the hand due to high-venous pressure; (2) arterial side to venous end, which is hard to perform, gives good blood flow, and results in the fewest complications; (3) arterial end to venous side and (4) arterial end to venous end, which result in low blood flow. It may take 1–3 months for the fistula to mature.

59. D: There are certain situations in which an arteriovenous fistula or graft is not immediately required or possible. In these cases, a central venous catheter threaded into a large thoracic vein usually provides enough blood flow to be feasible for dialysis. Patients with acute renal failure who may recover kidney function or those with drug overdoses are candidates for such blood access. Since it may take up to 3 months for a fistula to mature enough to be a reliable blood access site, dialysis may be started while waiting for the fistula to mature. Some patients have extensively damaged vessels from surgery or vascular disease, which precludes direct vascular access. Some patients waiting for a peritoneal catheter or a live donor kidney may also be maintained by a central catheter.

60. A: A graft is created by the surgical connection of an artery and vein, using an artificial vessel. Several different types of graft material are available. Grafts allow access to large volumes of blood but are more prone to complications than fistulae since they are "foreign" to the body. These grafts are more prone to stenosis (narrowing) of the vessels and clotting since the graft material may activate the blood coagulation and hemostatic mechanisms. Grafts tend to be more prone to infection and have a shorter useful lifespan than fistulae (less than 5 years on average). However grafts may be used in situations where native vessels are inadequate for fistula surgery.

61. C: Part of the technician's job is to evaluate the fistula site for problems and gauge its maturity. Annulations of the fistula is usually done by a nurse or physician. Technicians should check for evidence of infection, such as erythema, tenderness, fluctuation, or purulent drainage. Healing of the surgical incision should also be noted as incomplete healing may lead to infection. A thrill should be felt over the mature fistula as a continuous vibration, not a discrete pulsation as in an artery. A bruit may also be heard over the fistula site with a stethoscope. Application of a tourniquet and palpation of the fistula vein offers an index of its development as the vein thickens. One authority states that if access development is not seen by 2 weeks after surgery, it may not mature.

62. A: Sterile technique must be used before cannulating the blood access site. Hand washing and sterile gloves are mandatory. Preparation of the site should be carried out by application of the antiseptic in an outward circular motion from the site of needle insertion to avoid spreading bacteria toward the site. Four different antiseptic solutions are commonly used, the choice of which is determined by the particular dialysis center. Note that 70% alcohol alone is able to kill bacteria when wet so needle insertion requires only a short waiting period until the alcohol dries. Longer waiting periods are applicable to the other common antiseptics, which kill bacteria when dry: 3–5 minutes for Betadine, 30 seconds for ChloraPrep, and 2 minutes for Except Plus.

63. B: The most common arteriovenous fistula links the radial artery to the cephalic vein in the forearm. Another, though less frequent, arteriovenous link is in the upper arm, using the brachial artery and the cephalic vein. Other possible anastamoses include use of the ulnar artery linked to the basilar vein in the medial forearm or the femoral artery connected to the great saphenous vein in the thigh. Sometimes the normal anatomic course of the vessel must be surgically altered to bring it in proximity to the connecting vessel. For arm fistulae the blood flow to the hand must be checked. Arteriovenous fistulae may increase the cardiac workload by 10% so that patients with heart failure may not be good candidates. Veins must in good anatomical shape as well as long and straight to facilitate multiple needle sites.

64. C: Before inserting a needle into the access site, a look, feel, and listen approach should be taken. This includes checking for visual signs of infection or low blood flow to the hand (i.e., pale, bluish nail beds or skin). The access site should also be checked for scabs, flats spots, aneurysms (i.e., ballooning of the vessel), and stenosis (i.e., swollen access arm, pale skin, small blue or purple veins on the chest wall where the arm meets the body). A stethoscope is used to check for a bruit. Skin temperature should be neither too warm nor cold compared with the contralateral side. One should feel for a thrill and identify possible sites for needle insertion, avoiding previous sites of cannulation and staying 1.5 inches from the anastamosis.

65. C: Proper insertion of the dialysis needles is an acquired skill requiring patience and practice. Some patients will be more difficult than others. Always use a tourniquet high on the access arm even if it does not seem required; be sure to remove it before dialysis begins. Aim the needle at an angle consistent with the depth of the vessel, bevel up. Usually correct placement is indicated by a fall in resistance and blood flashback into the needle hub. Arterial and venous needles should be 1.5–2.0 inches apart. The venous needle should always be inserted in an antegrade direction (in the direction of the blood flow) and is downstream from the arterial needle. The arterial needle may be inserted in either antegrade or retrograde fashion. Once inserted the needle should not be rotated since this may tear the vessel wall or cause infiltration.

66. A: The buttonhole technique of needle insertion uses the same needle access point repeatedly. It has been found to lessen the incidence of infections, hematomas, and infiltrations. The concept is to use a sharp needle at the same angle and the same holes in the vessel until a scar tunnel (track) forms. Old scabs over insertion sites must be removed first; this can be done, using alcohol pads and sterile forceps. Once the tunnel is formed, a blunt needle is used in the same spots to avoid injuring the tunnel wall and causing leakage during dialysis. A scar tunnel takes about 3-4 weeks to form. Both arterial and venous needles should be inserted in an antegrade fashion (in the direction of blood flow) to enhance hemostasis after needle removal.

67. D: One in ten patients have a fear (phobia) of needles or blood, and a so-called vasovagal reaction may occur. This is characterized by a brief rise in pulse rate and blood pressure followed by a marked slowing of the pulse and a drop in blood pressure. The latter often leads to sweating, dizziness, and fainting. Preventive measures include recumbent posture rather than sitting during needle insertion; tensing the muscles of the nonaccess limbs for 10–20 seconds, relaxing and then repeating while the needle is being inserted; teaching the patient to insert his or her own needles, preferably using the buttonhole technique; and avoiding the pain of needle insertion by distraction (listening to music, watching television) or skin stretching by the so-called three-point technique. Local anesthetic (e.g., lidocaine), topical anesthetic, or ethyl chloride spray may also lessen the pain of needle insertion.

68. B: The term recirculation refers to dialyzed blood (venous) mixing with blood entering the arterial needle. Already dialyzed blood goes through the dialyzer again so less new blood is cleaned. Recirculation leads to a less efficient dialysis and may cause persistent symptoms of uremia. It may occur when the blood flow in the dialyzer is greater than in the arteriovenous fistula, when arterial and venous needles are placed too close together, when the arterial and venous lines are reversed, or when a stenosis is present. Major recirculation may lead to deoxygenation of the blood, the so-called "black blood" syndrome. If recirculation is suspected, the fistula is palpated to determine the direction of blood flow, and the needles are placed at least 1.5 inches apart.

69. A: When a fistula access diverts too much blood flowing into the hand, a so-called steal syndrome occurs. There is a relative lack of oxygen (hypoxia) to the hand, and symptoms, such as pain, tingling, numbness, or cold, may occur. Sometimes bluish nail beds or necrotic spots appear. Diabetic patients and others with compromised vasculature are most susceptible. The steal syndrome usually diminishes with time since collateral vessels develop that oxygenate the hand. Keeping the hand warm with a mitten or hand warmer and changing the arm position to take advantage of gravitational force may improve symptoms. Up to 5% of patients with arteriovenous fistulas may have steal syndrome, but it can be relieved by decreasing the blood flow through the fistula or surgically modifying the supply vessels.

70. D: Stenosis is a narrowing of the blood vessel conducting blood through the anastomosis. It reduces the blood flow and predisposes to thrombosis. The common sites are in the vein next to the anastomosis, a so-called juxta-anastomotic stenosis; anywhere along the course of the outflow vein, at a previous needle insertion site; or in a more central vein, particularly in the upper-shoulder region, possibly due to a previous central catheter. A high-pitched bruit, a water hammer pulse, diminished thrill, or difficulty inserting needles may all be signs of stenosis. There also may be increased venous pressure and swelling of the patient's access limb and an inability to obtain the prescribed blood flow rate. Some stenoses may be treated with angioplasty, while others require surgical revision.

71. C: Thrombosis (blood clot) may form in any vascular access device but is least common in an arteriovenous fistula. This may be because the blood is not exposed to a foreign substance that activates the hemostatic-coagulation cascade. However turbulence, low blood flow, stenosis or compression of the vessel, or damage to the vascular wall all predispose to thrombosis. Heparin anticoagulation is usually employed during dialysis Other maneuvers to diminish the risk of thrombosis during the periods between dialyses are to instruct patients to: not use the access site for routine blood drawing, drug administration, or intravenous lines; self-cannulate; not sleep on the access arm or carry heavy items with it; and not put too much pressure on the site after removal of the needles.

72. B: High-output cardiac failure may be seen in patients with anemia, hyperthyroidism, or arteriovenous shunts. The latter increases the venous return to the heart (by 20% or more), increasing the cardiac workload and decreasing the arterial resistance. Tachycardia and hypotension may occur. Symptoms of heart failure, such as dyspnea (shortness of breath) and peripheral edema, will ensue. Often patients with end stage renal disease are anemic or have coexisting heart disease, which worsens the problem. Treating anemia to hemoglobin levels above 10–11 g/dL and perhaps use of inotropic (heart contraction stimulants) drugs may help. Because the kidneys are not functional, diuretics are not useful. Reducing fluid gain between dialyses and removing more fluid by longer or more frequent dialyses may also be beneficial.

73. B: Arteriovenous grafts have certain advantages over fistulas, but they may be outweighed by complications. Animal or human blood vessels have been used in the past but are rarely used currently. Most commonly synthetic materials, such as collagen or expanded polytetrafluoroethylene, are used. Synthetic grafts may be straight or looped and usually offer a longer site for needle cannulation than fistulas. Common forearm straight grafts link the radial artery to the basilica vein, and loop grafts may link the brachial artery to the basilic vein. Most grafts require less time to mature than fistulas, but some graft materials may be cannulated immediately after insertion. Grafts may be useful in patients with vascular disease that renders a fistula unsuitable. The biggest problem with grafts is their tendency to infection and thrombosis, which exceeds that of fistulas. No synthetic graft material is as good as a native blood vessel from patients without vascular disease.

74. A: It is important that the dialysis technician does not choose a needle insertion site at the arterial or venous anastomosis; the placement should be at least 1 inch away, and the needles should be at least 2 inches apart. Needle puncture sites should be 0.25–0.5 inches away from a previous site. Needles may be placed along all three sides of the graft, not just on the top. One technique is to find the midpoint of the graft and then with each subsequent insertion the arterial needle is placed closer to the arterial anastomosis, and the venous needle is placed closer to the venous anastomosis. When the space limit is reached, the technician should start at the midpoint again. Needle direction should be antegrade for the venous side and antegrade or retrograde (preferred) for the arterial side.

75. C: Catheter-supported hemodialysis is used in a variety of situations, for example, when dialysis is anticipated to be temporary, when the patient refuses a fistula, when there is a wait for a scheduled transplant, or when there is an infected fistula or graft. The catheter is usually threaded into the large vessels of the chest and then into the right atrium or into the femoral vein and then into the inferior vena cava. The venous site must be able to support a high blood flow since it serves as both source and destination for the dialyzed blood. The best venous access is into the right internal jugular since it is a large vessel, is easily cannulated, and has a short and straight path into the right atrium. It has a low thrombosis rate as well. The second most preferable route is the left internal jugular, which is longer and has two curves so that blood flow tends to be slower. The femoral vein may be used for emergencies or if the neck veins are not available, but its position in the groin makes it less satisfactory for the patient. Subclavian veins should be used as a last resort.

76. D: Catheter infections are common and may lead to infection of the blood (sepsis). Rigorous adherence to sterile protocol should be the rule when catheters are opened or manipulated. The technician should wash hands and don sterile gloves. Most authorities demand wearing of masks by both the technician or nurse and the patient. Nasal and mouth bacteria are potential pathogens so both orifices should be covered. Dressings should be changed at each dialysis session. If the dressing gets wet, it should be replaced after drying the insertion site. Swimming or showering may be proscribed, but there are waterproof devices to keep catheter tips dry. The patient should be taught proper procedure for managing needle sticks or accidental cutting of the catheter.

77. C: If flow diminishes and a low-pressure alarm rings during catheter dialysis, the technician should first check for bleeding or air entry. Then the catheter position and integrity should be checked. The technician may also move the patient to a more recumbent posture or have him or her cough to reposition the catheter tip and possibly improve the flow. Flushing the line with saline is acceptable as well. Switching the lines so that the blood is pulled through the "venous" port and returned through the "arterial" port may help the problem, but it also causes recirculation and should only be done after checking with the nurse or supervising physician. A thrombolytic enzyme may be administered by either of these individuals. The arterial pre-pump and venous pressure gauges should be kept open since they relate the condition of both lumens.

78. C: Many patients favor catheters because they do not require needle sticks for access. The latter is usually done with connection of a syringe or tubing via a Luer-Lock adapter. The patient's arms and hands are free during the dialysis, and he or she can swim or shower with port/catheter devices once the incision is healed and stitches are removed. Catheters also provide an immediate site for drug administration or blood transfusion in case of a life-threatening emergency. The major problems with catheter type blood access methods are the higher risk of infection, the increased chance of thrombosis, and the low flow over time.

79. A: Transferring patients from a wheelchair to the dialysis chair and back may be done by several different techniques, depending on the weight of the patient and his or her ability to bear weight and assist with the transfer. Patients who can stand by themselves may be transferred by a single person, using the stand and pivot technique. This requires the use of a canvas belt around the patient's waist to assist standing then the patient is pivoted and lowered into the dialysis chair. The belt is then removed. A chair-to-chair transfer from a sitting position may be done, using a slide board. Two additional people are needed: one to help the patient as he or she slides on the board and another to lock and hold the wheelchair. For heavy patients unable to assist in the transfer, a portable lift device is preferable. This maneuver requires at least two staff people, one to move the lift and another to adjust the patient to the correct position in the dialysis chair.

80. C: A dialysis center should have emergency procedures that all staff members must know. Often procedures are posted on a wall in plain sight so that forgetting is less likely. In case of fire, if small, the proper sequence is RACE: rescue patients, activate the alarm, contain the fire, and evacuate the premises. Small fires may be controlled by a fire extinguisher: pull the pin, aim the nozzle at the base of the flames, pull the handle or trigger, and spray the base of the fire from side to side. Patients who can walk on their own may be disconnected from the dialysis machine and evacuated first. Patients who require some assistance and those who cannot walk will require staff help. While smoke inhalation is a problem in most fires in a contained space, rapid evacuation is preferable to using respirator masks. Once the alarm is sent, do not wait for the fire department before evacuating.

81. D: Aseptic technique is essential in manipulating the lines and syringes used on dialysis patients. Failure to do so increases the risk of infection, the second leading cause of death in these patients. Washing hands and using sterile gloves are standard procedures. Prepackaged sterile material should not get wet; these packages should be opened only when they are about to be used since they will be exposed to airborne pathogens. Touching a sterile item with a contaminated item contaminates it, and it should not then be used. The outside of a saline bag or medication vial should not be touched with a sterile needle. The ports should be scrubbed with 70% alcohol or other disinfectant. The ends of medication-filled syringes or the end of lines to and from the patient (e.g., heparin line) should not be touched.

82. C: One must change sterile gloves after each patient contact, when they have touched contaminated surfaces, or after handling infectious waste containers. Avoiding body fluids or blood is best done by wearing a gown, especially when putting in needles and injecting medication. Similarly, a face mask may protect against the spraying of potentially contaminated material to the eyes. Recapping needles or other sharps is dangerous, and needle sticks may transmit disease to staff members. If needle recapping must be done, use of a mechanical recapping device or one-handed technique is highly recommended. Sharps should be disposed in colored puncture-proof containers.

83. A: Hepatitis B is quite contagious and is transmitted by infected blood. A vaccine is available, and staff members and selected patients should receive it. Fresh external venous and arterial transducer protectors should be used for each treatment, and a separate room with a dedicated dialysis machine should be used for patients who test positive for hepatitis B surface antigen. Hepatitis C is also transmitted by infected blood but is less transmissible than hepatitis B so that dedicated dialysis machines are not required, and a separate room is unnecessary. HIV may be transmitted by blood and other body fluids; it is most often transmitted by sexual contact or shared needles by infected addicts in the general population. Isolation and dedicated machines are not required if standard infection control procedures are followed. Tuberculosis is spread by airborne droplets from sneezing or coughing by an infected person with active disease. It usually requires prolonged, close contact with the source to transmit the disease, but some cases have been reported in dialysis centers.

84. C: Medication for injection comes in a variety of vial sizes and concentrations. Reading the label several times during the withdrawal process is very important since drugs may have similar names and come in different concentrations. The expiration date should also be checked. Cleaning the rubber cap with disinfectant before withdrawal is mandatory. Injecting air equivalent to the volume to be withdrawn is a good practice for a multidose vial. Single-use vials may be discarded in an appropriate disposal container. Air bubbles should be expelled from the syringe by tapping the barrel to bring the air next to the needle as the syringe is held in a needle-up position and then gently pushing on the plunger to remove the air. If sterile technique is followed, there is no need to change needles during withdrawal.

85. B: Charting entries may be printed or in script but must be legible and in ink. Each entry must be followed by the writer's name and title. The standard method for corrections prohibits erasures or correction fluid. The error must have a single line through it, a written notation "error" or "mistake," and followed by initials of the writer. Abbreviations are discouraged since others may not be aware of their meaning, or one abbreviation may indicate more than one term. Most centers allow the use of approved abbreviations of which all staff members are familiar. Many centers are now using electronic charting. Passwords must be kept confidential, even from other staff members, and backup files are essential. Unauthorized persons are not allowed to view medical data, and printouts should be protected from prying eyes.

86. D: The estimated dry weight for the dialysis patient refers to the weight the patient should be with no excess fluid and a normal blood pressure. Based on the physician's estimate, the amount of fluid to remove during dialysis is calculated. It should be noted that not all weight gain between dialysis sessions is due to fluid accumulation. Some may be due to eating more, exercise with weights, or wearing different clothing. In general, patients who are below dry weight after treatment may be hypotensive or have postural (orthostatic) hypotension and dizziness when standing up. Muscle cramping is common in these patients. Edema, hypertension, and dyspnea suggest the patient is above the dry weight and may need further treatment.

87. D: Checking alarms of the extracorporeal circuit and dialysate is critical before treatment is begun. Alarms for the air detector, blood leak detector, arterial and venous high/low alarms must all be functioning. If any one of these alarms registers values outside the set limits, the pump will stop, and the venous line will clamp; the audio alarm will go off, and a visual message will appear. The dialysate alarms for conductivity, pH, and temperature must also be checked. If any of these go off, the dialysate flow goes into bypass mode, and flow to the dialyzer stops. In addition, tests should be done to insure that all germicide has been removed from the reprocessed dialyzer.

88. C: Taking pulse and blood pressure readings from the patient before dialysis are mandatory. Many dialysis machines can record the blood pressure, and there are numerous automatic devices now in use; however, technicians should know how and where to take it manually, using a stethoscope and sphygmomanometer (blood pressure cuff). The extremity should be at heart level (right atrium) when the pressure is taken to avoid higher (below the heart) or lower (above the heart) readings. In patients whose arms are not accessible or have lines inserted, blood pressure may be taken in the leg. Possible sites are in the thigh with the stethoscope over the popliteal artery or the calf with the stethoscope over the posterior tibial artery. It is important that the cuff is of adequate size, the bladder length 80% of the site circumference and the width 40% (arm or leg), according to the American Heart Association.

89. A: The patient's vital signs— pulse rate, blood pressure, temperature, and respiratory rate— must be taken and recorded. Many centers also include a pulse oximetry value; normal is usually 95% or higher. For a young adult, pulse readings should be regular and between 60–100/min.

Blood pressure is considered elevated if the reading is greater than 140 systolic or 90 diastolic. Many authorities believe that the systolic pressure should be below 130 for diabetic patients. A drop of 15 mm Hg or more on standing from a sitting position is called orthostatic hypotension and may cause dizziness or fainting. Temperature for young adults is 98.6°F (37°C) and somewhat lower for the elderly. Most authorities consider temperatures above 100°F (37.8°C) as fever. A normal respiratory rate is usually 12–16 breaths/min.

90. D: Most volumetric dialysis machines can calculate and set the appropriate pressures and hourly ultrafiltration rate for fluid removal. However, the technician must still calculate the volume of fluid to be removed and set the duration of dialysis. The difference between the patient's current weight and estimated dry weight with 1 K = 1000 mL is added to the saline prime, the rinse back volume (volume of saline used to push blood back into patient after dialysis stopped), and the volume of any medications or fluids given during treatment (e.g., food, ice chips, drinks). Fluid output in the form of urine (if any) or vomiting is not usually used in the calculation.

91. B: Drawing blood samples from the patient is a routine part of any dialysis program. The blood should be drawn from the arterial port or arterial tubing before giving heparin or saline. Blood tests are usually drawn before treatment except postdialysis blood urea nitrogen, recirculation studies, or blood cultures. All blood tests must be ordered by a physician or by a physician-approved protocol. Blood for anticoagulant free tubes (e.g., red top) should be drawn before those in which there is anticoagulant (e.g., purple top). A small amount of blood drawn from a catheter must be discarded before obtaining the sample. The line may then be cleared with saline. Blood tubes should not be placed on a warm surface as hemolysis or alteration of the laboratory test may result.

92. A: The urea reduction ratio (URR) is an estimate of the amount of urea removed by dialysis. Urea is a small, easily measured molecule and is a chief waste product, requiring excretion by the kidneys. The URR is usually determined by measuring the pre- and post-dialysis blood urea nitrogen (BUN), using the following formula: URR (%) = 100[1–(BUNpost/BUNpre)]. While the URR is a useful measure of the effectiveness of dialysis, it has its limitations. If low, it does not inform you how much extra time for dialysis is needed. It does not account for the amount of urea formed during dialysis or the amount removed by ultrafiltration. For the latter, a more complex calculation called urea kinetic modeling is required. This provides the above information and takes into account the patient's size and residual kidney function.

93. C: The urea kinetic modeling (UKM) calculation can be used for both prescribed doses for the patient and the actual amount delivered. The formula is Kt/V, where K is the urea clearance in mL/min, t is the time of dialysis, and V is the volume of urea in the patient's body. According to renal disease authorities, the minimum delivered dose should be a Kt/V of 1.2 (URR approximately 65%), and the minimum prescribed dose should be a Kt/V of 1.4 (urea reduction ratio, approximately 70%). Pre- and post-dialysis blood urea nitrogen measurements are required with the blood samples drawn at the same session. The K value depends on the dialyzer, blood, and dialysate flow rates. The value of V is hard to measure, and a computer program is used for its estimation.

94. C: Priming the reprocessed dialyzer removes the germicide before patient use. The dialyzer blood compartment should be primed with normal saline, followed by flushing the dialysate compartment. Ensure air is removed from the arterial line before it is attached to the dialyzer to avoid pushing air into the extracorporeal circuit and the dialyzer. 300-400 mL (or per manufacturer's instructions) of normal saline must be primed through the dialyzer. This should be done at a low blood pump speed to minimize turbulence. This is because peracetic acid can form gas bubbles when exposed to buffered dialysate. The bubbles can cause clotting in the dialyzer fibers and prevent the total elimination of peracetic acid from the dialyzer. Testing for residual germicide MUST be performed immediately prior to initiating treatment. A minimum of two people must verify the negative test result prior to treatment initiation, including the patient if appropriate.

95. D: Heparin administration is standard during dialysis to prevent blood clotting. The dose is usually adjusted to double the activated clotting time of the blood; some centers use a laboratory-determined partial thromboplastin time. Some patients cannot receive heparin because of excessive bleeding, allergic reactions, or a history of heparin-induced thrombocytopenia. For patients who have only minor bleeding (i.e., skin ecchymoses, nosebleed, access site oozing), a lower dose of heparin may suffice. Warfarin, a vitamin K–inhibiting anticoagulant, is usually given orally and has too slow an onset and too prolonged an offset for use in dialysis. Regional citrate anticoagulation is rarely used but may be useful in those who cannot take heparin. Trisodium citrate is infused into the arterial line to remove calcium ions, which prevents clotting; the calcium is then restored by giving calcium chloride into the venous line.

96. A: Bacterial infections are fairly common in dialysis patients and must be recognized and treated promptly. A purulent discharge at the exit site of a catheter is most likely to be due to *Staphylococcus aureus,* which is present on the skin and mucous membranes. Many strains are so-called methicillin-resistant *Staph. aureus* (MRSA), which indicates that they are resistant to many antibiotics. Because this organism may cause sepsis, pneumonia, or other life-threatening infections, strict adherence to aseptic technique and prompt use of an antibiotic to which the organism is sensitive are mandatory. *Enterococcus* is a bacterium that lives in the gastrointestinal tract but may spread elsewhere and be hard to eradicate, especially the vancomycin-resistant strains. *Clostridioides difficile* is another gastrointestinal organism that may proliferate, especially during or after antibiotic therapy, and secrete a harmful toxin. *Mycoplasma* rarely causes skin infections but may be the causative agent of community-acquired pneumonia.

97. B: Anaphylactic reactions are severe allergic reactions that may be caused by residual germicide in the dialysis tubing (e.g., ethylene oxide) or drugs, such as heparin, iron dextran, or certain antibiotics. The pattern is one of dyspnea, often due to laryngeal spasm; hives; itching; and hypotension. This is a medical emergency and requires immediate treatment with epinephrine, steroids, and antihistamine plus vascular support. An air embolus from a broken connection in the extracorporeal circuit or empty intravenous bag may cause chest pain, dyspnea, and cyanosis but not itching or hives. Angina is also a potential cause of dyspnea and chest pain, as many patients have a history of coronary artery disease with episodes of angina; however, hives and itching are unusual; Sublingual nitroglycerin spray or tablets may be used. Disequilibrium syndrome is characterized by neurologic symptoms in reaction to rapid removal of urea from the blood, resulting in water entry into the brain.

98. C: Removal of too much fluid during the dialysis procedure may induce muscle cramps, especially in the hands, arms, and feet. Dehydration leads to electrolyte imbalance, especially hypernatremia that results in severe muscular cramping. Low-potassium levels (hypokalemia) may also result in muscle cramps. Low-calcium levels are more likely to cause myalgias and muscle spasms than hypercalcemia. Hypotension may also be a cause of muscle cramps. Preventive measures include obtaining the patient's correct weight, calculating the correct volume of fluid to be removed, checking and using the prescribed dialysate concentrate, and reviewing the salt and fluid dietary limits with the patient.

99. D: Hemolysis, rupturing of the red blood cell membrane and releasing hemoglobin and other contents, may be caused by trauma to the cells, hypotonic solutions, high temperature, immune reactions, and direct injury by chemicals. The remains of the cell are referred to as ghosts. Kinked bloodlines may be a traumatic cause. Inadequate water treatment that allows chloramines, copper, zinc, or nitrates into the dialysate may also cause hemolysis. Dialysate at too high a temperature will cause hemolysis as will residual formaldehyde in a reused dialyzer. If too much hemoglobin is released into the patient's circulation, nausea, headache, back pain, and changes in blood pressure can occur. Additional kidney damage may occur. A centrifuged blood sample will show a red supernatant serum. The dialysate conductivity and temperature should be checked and tested for chloramines and disinfectants. Bloodlines should be inspected for kinking.

100. C: After each treatment, bloodline tubing and all other disposable equipment should be discarded. Many centers use disposable dialyzers. For reprocessing, heparinized saline should be circulated through the dialyzer to remove blood, making sure there is no air in the circuit, which promotes residual clotting. A dialyzer that is to be reused should be refrigerated or reprocessed within 10–15 minutes of its last use. Clamps and the outside of the dialysis machine should be chemically disinfected. The dialysate delivery system must also be disinfected, using a hot water (85°C–95°C) recirculation method or a chemical disinfectant. In the latter, the rinse water washes out the disinfectant but must be tested for residual disinfectant.

101. A: Reusing dialyzers reduces hypersensitivity reactions, including anaphylactic symptoms. A reaction in the first 15–30 minutes with the use of a new dialyzer is not uncommon. Most reactions are due to sensitization to ethylene oxide, which is used to sterilize most new dialyzers in the United States. Repeated rinsing lowers the level of the germicide so that reactions are less common with reused dialyzers. Some centers prefer to reuse dialyzers since there may be a more efficient removal of middle-sized molecules, such as $beta_2$-globulin. This is particularly true for the expensive high-flux dialyzers. The preponderance of evidence indicates that reuse of dialyzers does not lead to an increased patient mortality. Reuse also saves money and reduces medical waste.

102. B: Reuse of dialyzers must be done according to Association for the Advancement of Medical Instrumentation standards. These have also been adopted by the Centers for Medicare and Medicaid Services as a condition for coverage for dialysis centers. These guidelines cover the type of equipment, cleaning, and disinfecting, water use for reprocessing, labeling, and also staff training and standards. Each dialyzer type must be labeled for single or multiple use. Not all germicides may be used in all dialyzers; the manufacturer must specify. There are also rules relating to required equipment, environmental safety, and quality assurance. Reprocessing may be done manually or by machine, but the latter, automated process is considered more efficient.

103. C: Before initial use, a new dialyzer should be checked for its baseline total cell volume (TCV), also called fiber bundle volume. TCV measures the amount of solute and ultrafiltration for the dialyzer's next use. The TCV or baseline clearance (e.g., urea, sodium, ionic clearance) should be measured after each reprocessing and compared to the previous value for that machine. Different dialyzers have different TCV and clearance values so batch comparisons may not be valid. Preprocessing of new dialyzers is done at many centers to remove potentially noxious substances and to obtain an accurate TCV. Each dialyzer must be labeled with the patient's name and identification data; number, date, and time of use; the name or identification of the reprocessing staff member; and the results of any tests done on the dialyzer.

104. A: The initial step after completion of the dialysis treatment is to rinse the blood in the dialyzer back to the patient. This avoids additional patient blood loss and improves the dialyzer's performance if it is to be reused. If rinse back is poor, the dialyzer should be discarded. The dialyzer is then disconnected from the extracorporeal circuit and subjected to precleaning in the reprocessing room. The latter may be done by reverse ultrafiltration. Germicides may be used during the precleaning process. The total cell volume or clearance must then be measured, according to federal regulations. A test for blood leaks is also mandatory. Cracks or a defect in the dialyzer's plastic housing is another reason to discard it.

105. B: After cleaning, the structure and function of the dialyzer must be tested if it is to be reused. A few or no streaks of blood indicate a good rinse back, but those with many streaks should not be reused. Recommendations by renal authorities state that dialyzers with less than 90% of their original clearance value (e.g., urea, sodium, ionic) or less than 80% of their original total cell volume should not be reused. Additional reasons to discard dialyzers are: it has reached its maximal number of uses (per center policy); it has cracks or other defects in the plastic housing; it has blood leaks; it has been exposed to more than one germicide; or it has many discolored fibers.

106. D: Germicides are used to kill pathogens. No more than one type may be used during reprocessing. There are four main germicides in use in the United States: peracetic acid (the most common), formaldehyde, glutaraldehyde, and heat. All have minimum contact periods with the dialyzer; for example, peracetic acid must remain in contact for 11 hours and formaldehyde for 24 hours. Each germicide has good and bad features. Peracetic acid breaks down to water, oxygen, and acetic acid (relatively harmless and biodegradable) but is expensive. Formaldehyde, though cheap, has many potentially toxic effects on the technician and requires a long contact period. Heat is free of toxic or environmental effects and is cheap but is not compatible with all dialyzers. Glutaraldehyde is also inexpensive but can potentially cause skin and respiratory problems in the technician.

107. C: Bacteria and endotoxin may enter the dialysate. A common source is the water used to make the dialysate. The endotoxin is a lipopolysaccharide or lipooligosaccharide portion of the bacterial cell wall and has immunogenic properties. It is present in the outer membrane of certain gram-negative bacteria and may cause pyrogenic reactions or septic shock in the patient if it enters the blood. Both bacteria and endotoxin may be adsorbed to the housing, support structure, and membranes of the dialyzer. Use of outdated germicides or inadequate exposure time may allow bacterial growth. The Association for the Advancement of Medical Instrumentation has established standards for bacterial and endotoxin concentration in the reprocessing water: less than 200 bacterial colony forming units and less than 2 endotoxin units/mL. If there is a pyrogenic reaction or septicemia, the center must stop reprocessing and must evaluate the entire process.

108. C: Federal regulations require proof that a center can safely reprocess dialyzers. There are two components to this required program. Quality assurance indicates that all policies and procedures regarding reuse have been recorded and are being followed. These standards are quite detailed and are available from the American Association of Medical Instrumentation. Quality control refers to meeting the set standards of the reprocessing procedure, for example total cell volume measurement, tests for bacteria and endotoxin, and tests for the presence or absence of germicide. If done correctly, dialyzer reprocessing may be carried out safely and with confidence that no harm will come to patients. However if done incorrectly, a variety of problems may arise; anaphylactic symptoms, sleep problems, damage to the immune system, respiratory distress, and burning in the vascular access are some of the untoward events.

109. D: Water is required to make dialysate, to mix concentrate, and to flush out and reprocess the dialyzer. Rainwater typically acquires contaminants during its passage through the atmosphere (e.g., carbon dioxide, sulfur dioxide), which result in acid formation. Ground water from springs or wells dissolves numerous chemical compounds, such as nitrates, sodium, chloride, magnesium salts, and iron. Surface water from lakes and rivers is usually higher in sewage and bacterial contamination and pesticides. Normal kidneys may eliminate many contaminants from tap water that is imbibed, but contaminants must be removed from water used for dialysis. Calcium carbonate is the most common impurity in tap water. Many substances added to tap water to make it safer (e.g., chloramine, fluoride, alum) are potentially harmful to the dialysis patient and must be removed by a water treatment process.

110. C: A healthy individual drinks between 10–14 liters a week, and the amount retained depends on functioning kidneys and a complex system of baroreceptors and hormones (e.g., antidiuretic hormone). The average dialysis patient receives 350 L a week (270–576 liters) in the dialysate. Such a large volume exposes the patient to much higher amounts of contaminants. Improperly treated water may cause a variety of problems, such as nausea, vomiting, hemolysis, anemia, marked changes in blood pressure, and even death. The American Association of Medical Instrumentation water treatment standards for water to be used for dialysis include maximum levels for bacteria, endotoxin, metals, salts, trace elements, and other potentially toxic substances.

111. C: Water must be purified for dialysis. This usually requires a series of components to eliminate bacteria and harmful chemicals. The component placement in the treatment cycle is referred to as upstream or downstream with reference to another component. Water must be kept in motion to avoid bacterial growth. After tapping purified water for the dialysate, there is a recycling system so that the residual water is returned to the purifying pathway. This saves water and prevents stagnant spots. Seasonal changes in water contaminants and local variations in bacterial or chemical impurities must be taken into account for the design and operation of an efficient water treatment system.

112. D: One-way circulation in the water treatment system is maintained by a backflow prevention device that prevents water and possible contaminants from returning to the feed source. Water temperature must be maintained at 77°F–82°F (25°C–28°C) to prevent reduction in the efficiency of the reverse osmosis membrane downstream. There is a 1.5% decrease in this membrane for every 1°F decrease in temperature. The temperature adjustment is accomplished with a blending valve that mixes hot and cold water and a thermometer downstream to monitor the actual temperature. In case there is a fall in water pressure from the source, a booster pump may be placed downstream from the temperature blending valve with pressure gauges before and after the pump.

113. B: Feed water should have a pH in the 5.0–8.5 range before further treatment. If the water has a higher pH (more basic) then acids (e.g., hydrochloric or sulfuric) may be added to bring the pH down into the acceptable range. Similarly, chloramines may be reduced by adding sodium bisulfite to the feed water. The chemical addition component must have a reservoir to hold the chemical, a metering pump to deliver the correct amount of chemical, and a mixing chamber to distribute the added chemical effectively into the feed water line. Sodium hydroxide is a strong base and would raise the pH.

114. A: Sediment filters remove particles and some solutes by straining. Usually there is a progression of filters with smaller and smaller pores so that small-sized particles are successively filtered out. The multimedia filter may contain a 5-micron filter to screen out large particles and successively smaller submicron filters (e.g., 0.01 micron) to eliminate small particulate matter. Trapped particles may clog the pores of the filter. One way of managing this is to recirculate water from the bottom of the filter to the top to clean the filters and remix the water. This is called backwashing and should be carried out when the system is not in use. An ultrafilter, which is able to trap very small particles, including bacteria, may be placed further downstream.

115. A: Hard water contains many minerals, including calcium and magnesium, that precipitate out and form scale. These metals are usually removed by an ion exchange process in a so-called water softener. This exchange takes place on a bed of polystyrene beads coated with sodium chloride ions. The sodium is exchanged for calcium and magnesium ions, which are also positively charged. When the resin is saturated with calcium and magnesium, it must be regenerated and again coated with sodium ions. This is done by flushing the resin with water and then with brine (concentrated sodium chloride). The calcium and magnesium exchange with the fresh sodium and are washed into a drain. Regeneration must not be done during dialysis so that a highly concentrated sodium solution is not presented to the reverse osmosis membrane downstream. Adsorption, filtration, and osmosis do not play a role in water softening by ion exchange.

116. B: Carbon tanks contain granular activated charcoal (GAC) not powdered charcoal, which efficiently adsorbs chlorine, chloramine, and other organic substances and solvents. It requires two tanks in series: an initial "worker" and a second "polisher." There must be enough exposure time to the charcoal to remove the chemicals effectively, the so-called empty bed contact time. This is usually 10 minutes or 5 minutes for each tank. A 12 x 40 or smaller carbon mesh size should be used, and the GAC should have an iodine rating (i.e., that measures the efficiency of adsorption) of greater than 900. Backwashing of the charcoal does not effectively remove the adsorbed chemicals so that the first tank is replaced by the second tank, and a fresh tank is added to replace the second.

117. C: In osmosis, water traverses a semipermeable membrane to equalize the solute concentration or until hydrostatic pressure equalizes the osmotic pressure. In reverse osmosis, hydrostatic pressure derived from a pump is used to drive water through the membrane, leaving concentrated solute and organic material greater than 200 microns to be flushed into the drain or recycled back to the input of the reverse osmotic system. Prefilters are used just before the reverse osmotic system to screen out any residual particulate matter. These must be changed on a regular basis. The membranes are thin film composites made of polyamide. The membranes must be cleaned every 4 months and disinfected with 1% peracetic acid monthly.

118. C: Deionization removes cations (positively charged ions) and anions (negatively charged ions) from water but does not remove particles that are not charged. Electrically charged resin beads exchange hydrogen ions (H^+) for cations and hydroxyl ions (OH^-) for anions, producing water (H_2O). So-called dual-bed tanks contain either cation or anion resin beads, while mixed-bed tanks contain both anion and cation resin beads. Mixed bed tanks produce purer water than the dual tanks. Portable tanks are used but must be regenerated off-site. Caution is required so that industrial-grade resins are not used as these contain numerous contaminants; medical- or food-grade resins are required. Exhaustion of the resin is a potential problem so the tank size should be specified and monitored carefully.

119. A: An ultraviolet irradiator may be used in some water treatment systems to destroy bacteria. Light at a wavelength of 254 nanometers is emitted by a mercury lamp. This light alters the bacterial DNA so it dies or cannot multiply. The water flows through a sleeve made of quartz material that admits light. Flow limits are indicated by the manufacturer. Newer systems have a radiation-dose monitor that registers when the bulb needs replacing and sets off an alarm. The quartz sleeve also requires periodic cleaning. The irradiator is usually placed after the carbon tanks but before the reverse osmosis component to decrease the bacterial concentration of water entering the latter.

120. D: A biofilm is an aggregate of microorganisms in which cells adhere to each other or to surfaces. An extracellular polymeric substance (sometimes called slime) is produced by the organisms and changes their growth pattern. The latter may be different from the plankton (single-cell form) of the same organism. It is a common problem in hospitals or dialysis center water treatment equipment and very hard to remove. Triggering factors for the switch to a biofilm growth pattern include availability of surface attachment sites, nutritional factors, or exposure to subinhibitory concentrations of antibiotics. Disinfectant of the water treatment system may be done with bleach, heat, or ozone, but substantial biofilm adherence may require complete replacement of the conduits.

121. B: In 1972, Congress passed Public Law 92-603, which covered dialysis and kidney transplants for patients with end-stage renal disease. It established a Medicare coverage provision for all those entitled to Social Security based on their employment, some 93% of patients. The Medicare contribution is 80% of allowable costs, while the balance is paid by private insurance, state support, or the patient. Subsequently, employer group insurance was made the primary payer for the initial 30 months of treatment (average payment is $126,000/patient/year) while Medicare became the secondary payer (average of $63,000/year). Today's dialysis centers are paid a composite rate for each treatment by Medicare. This rate is based on the patient's weight, height, and age and does not automatically increase by an annual cost of living adjustment. Congress sets any rate increase.

122. A: About two-thirds of the dialysis centers today are owned by large dialysis companies. Since the large organizations continue to buy additional independent centers, this fraction will increase. While much dialysis in the very early years was done at home and later became hospital based, most centers today are freestanding. In 1978, end-stage renal disease (ESRD) networks were established to oversee the quality of dialysis treatments. There are now eighteen of these, which cover one to six states each. For example, one network covers Hawaii and Northern California, another covers Southern California, and another covers only Texas. Each of these ESRD networks is under contract with Medicare to oversee quality, collect data, and provide a patient grievance conduit.

123. D: Numerous state and national organizations set the standards and oversee the quality of dialysis centers. Centers for Medicare and Medicaid Services (CMS) inspect dialysis centers through contracts with state health authorities, which determine their certification. Loss of certification may mean loss of Medicare funding. Inspections may be infrequent because of the large number of centers and government budgetary problems. The End-Stage Renal Disease (ESRD) Networks play a role, and the Food and Drug Administration sets dialysis guidelines and a mechanism for reporting faulty equipment or unexpected drug reactions. The Joint Commission on the Accreditation of Healthcare Organizations has established standards for hospital-based dialysis centers, and the Association for the Advancement of Medical Instrumentation has set standards for water treatment, dialysate preparation, and reprocessing of dialyzers. Clinical Practice Guidelines are published annually by the National Kidney Foundation in cooperation with CMS and ESRD Networks.

124. C: Continuous quality improvement (CQI) is a systematic audit or review to assess and improve clinical, technical, and organizational problems that may exist in a dialysis center. This may be instituted by management ("top down") or by staff ("bottom up"). One popular four-step schedule is: (1) identify improvement needs; (2) analyze the process; (3) identify root causes; and (4) implement the plan, do, check, and act cycle. Each of the major steps has substeps that further delineate the exact process by which the CQI is conducted (e.g., the four steps outlined in step 4). Purifying water, improving blood access, or filling in a checklist of clinical data may all present problems that a CQI may identify and correct. Solutions may be as complicated as replacing certain equipment or as simple as changing a technician's work hours.

125. D: Professionalism is defined by "exhibiting a courteous, conscientious, and business-like manner in the workplace." While politeness is mandatory and patient dignity is always to be maintained, the patient is there for medical treatment and is not a friend. Thus, first names or nicknames should not be used without request, and the technician should avoid discussing personal problems or plans with the patient. There is a temptation to make the patient feel more at ease or worry less if good results of other patients are shared, but this too should be avoided. All personal information concerning patients must be kept private, and the patient's medical or other problems must not be discussed with others as their privacy must be maintained. It is permissible to take a short break to talk with a patient calmly. Excessive shouting, running, or constant busyness may only add to the patient's anxiety.

126. A: The certified clinical hemodialysis technician examination (CCHT) requires completion of a training program for hemodialysis patient care technicians with both classroom instruction and supervised clinical work. Suggested but not required is 6-months of full-time or equivalent (1000 hours) experience, including training. This is an entry-level examination. There are additional examinations that require 12 months of clinical experience or completion of an approved course. For the CCHT, a high school diploma or GED and the signature of a preceptor or supervisor are also needed to document that the technician has received the appropriate training. One must also be in compliance with state regulations for clinical hemodialysis technicians.

127. B: The National Nephrology Certification Organization, Inc., gives two examinations for certification: one as a clinical nephrology technician (CCNT) and the other as a biomedical nephrology technician (CBNT). Both require at least 12 months of work experience. The CCNT examination measures knowledge in four areas: principles of dialysis, machine preparation and operation, patient assessment, and patient treatment. The CBNT examination assesses knowledge in six areas: principles of dialysis, scientific concepts, electronic applications, water treatment, equipment functions, and environmental/regulatory matters.

128. C: In 2003, the National Kidney Foundation issued a program entitled Kidney Disease: Improving Global Outcomes (KDIGO). This was a series of practice guidelines for patients with chronic kidney disease (CKD) worldwide. They included a number of problems associated with the condition and the suggested treatment. For example, anemia is a common feature of CKD, and the methods to ameliorate it are outlined: making sure dialysis patients receive more of their blood back after treatment, minimizing blood drawing for analysis or loss during needle sticks, and preventing clotting in the dialyzer. In addition, treatment with iron and erythropoietin indications are noted. KDIGO topics include dialysis dose and time, blood access, heart disease, high blood pressure, bone disease, lipid disorders, and other aspects of CKD.

129. C: Dialysis technicians often must lift equipment. Proper methods of lifting avoid back strain or other injury. Before lifting, the weight of the package or patient must be tested or assessed. If too heavy, assistance or use of a mechanical device must be requested. Most centers have mechanical lifts for patients and casters or dollies for moving heavy equipment. Good physical conditioning helps: ideal body weight, exercise, and flexibility all improve the ability to lift. Lifting should be done with the legs, holding the object close to the body. It is important not to twist and to lift at the same time. The feet, knees, and torso are pointed in the same direction, and asymmetric lifting should be avoided. Pushing an object is more effective than pulling.

130. D: One advantage of peritoneal dialysis (PD) is that there is more or less constant fluid in the abdomen; thus, the patient is exposed to more or less constant dialysis. It usually requires four or five exchanges of dialysate daily with so-called continuous ambulatory PD; however, a cycler that allows the process to be done at night during sleep (continuous cycling PD) is also quite popular. Since fluid is constantly in the abdomen, the dialysis duration is longer than in hemodialysis (HD), leading to less disequilibrium. Dietary restrictions may be lessened in PD. Fluid buildup is less of a problem in PD because it is within the abdomen and frequently exchanged. The biggest problem with PD is clogging or infection related to the intraperitoneal catheter. If an infection ensues, replacement may be required, and the patient must be maintained on HD in the interim.

131. D: In the past decade, the risk of death during or after a kidney transplant has been reduced to 3%–5% in the first year. This is not significantly different from patients on dialysis for the first year. These figures reflect death from any cause and are mostly related to complicating illnesses, such as diabetes; heart disease, especially coronary artery disease; chronic obstructive lung disease; and older age (older than 65). If the first transplant is rejected, there is a 10%–15% lower risk of success for a second transplant. Usually diseased kidneys are left in place during the transplant, although very high blood pressure or kidney infection may be grounds for removal.

132. B: Kidneys for transplantation are obtained from living relatives, live unrelated persons, and cadavers. These individual kidney donors undergo tissue and blood typing to check whether they are a match to the recipient. Virtually all kidney transplant patients receive immunosuppressive drugs to prevent rejection. Since they depress the immune system, infection may be a risk for any one of them. Despite this, only about 15% of transplant recipients have a serious infection. Cyclosporine combined with prednisone (a steroid) is often an initial combination given to these patients. Cyclosporine has renal toxicity and may cause a rise in the serum creatinine level. Dose reduction with blood level monitoring may be required. Steroids, such as prednisone, have a variety of immediate and long-term side effects, but since the post-transplant doses are usually low, they may be absent or tolerable. One noteworthy side effect is aggravation of diabetes so that patients previously on oral hypoglycemics may require insulin.

133. C: Potential kidney donors, whether living or cadavers, and possible recipients undergo numerous tests to determine compatibility of the kidney and the chance of rejection. A 6/6 human leukocyte antigen match and the same blood group offers the best chance of a successful transplant. This is most often a living relative, usually a sibling. A sensitization test is performed to detect potential serum antibodies of the recipient that might reject a donor kidney. The serum is tested again, a panel of lymphocytes are derived from multiple individuals, and the result is sometimes referred to as the panel reactive activity. The more highly reactive the recipient, the more difficult it is to find a suitable donor. If a potential donor is selected, the recipient serum is tested directly against the donor lymphocytes, a so-called crossmatch.

134. B: The kidneys play a major role in fluid and electrolyte balance, acid–base balance, waste excretion, and the production of erythropoietin. When renal failure occurs, waste, fluid, and certain ionic species tend to accumulate in the body. This may lead to hypertension, edema, metabolic acidosis, and pulmonary congestion. Potassium and phosphate tend to be retained so that foods rich in these substances should be limited. Phosphate elevation in the blood reduces the calcium level by forming calcium phosphate. Lowering of serum calcium stimulates the parathyroid glands to produce parathyroid hormone, so-called secondary hyperparathyroidism. This hormone increases calcium release from bone and may lead to weak, demineralized (osteoporotic) bone. Since the kidneys cannot excrete phosphate well in renal failure, phosphate binders are usually given to prevent hyperphosphatemia, and vitamin D is given to enhance calcium absorption.

135. D: The decision to begin hemodialysis in a patient with chronic renal failure is based on clinical and laboratory findings. Symptoms such as encephalopathy, seizures, or uremic coma are obvious indications for emergent hemodialysis. Other reasons may be pericarditis, acidosis, pulmonary edema unresponsive to medication, and hyperkalemia (elevated potassium), especially if the level is greater than 6.0 mEq/dL or if electrocardiographic changes are present. A creatinine clearance of 3–5 mL/min or a serum creatinine greater than 12–14 mg/dL are the usual laboratory indications. Most patients begin hemodialysis when conservative management fails to control symptoms or when abnormal laboratory values become worse despite appropriate treatment.

136. A: The nephrotic syndrome is a disorder in which the kidneys are damaged, usually by glomerular disease, which causes marked proteinuria (greater than 3.5 g/d/1.72 m² body surface area), hypoalbuminemia, hyperlipidemia, and edema due to the loss of albumin, ranging from facial puffiness to generalized edema (anasarca). Pleural effusion (fluid in the pleural space) and ascites (fluid in the abdomen) may occur. There are primary forms due to glomerular diseases, such as membranous nephropathy or focal segmental glomerulosclerosis and secondary forms caused by such diseases as diabetes mellitus, systemic lupus erythematosus, sarcoidosis, and amyloidosis or by drugs (steroids, gold). Hematuria (blood in the urine) is not usually a part of this syndrome.

137. B: Erythropoietin is a glycoprotein hormone released by the kidney in response to hypoxic stimuli. It stimulates the red cell precursors in the bone marrow to increase the rate of erythropoiesis to raise the red blood cell number (increases the hemoglobin concentration). The blood level of the hormone is elevated in polycythemia and low in chronic kidney disease (CKD). Several different commercial formulations are available for CKD patients on hemodialysis. It may be given subcutaneously or intravenously, preferably the latter into the venous line at the end of a dialysis session. Iron should also be given if the ferritin (iron storage protein) level is low. Current recommendations are to give the hormone to obtain a hemoglobin level of 10–12 g/dL. Higher levels may predispose to thrombosis. If the hemoglobin level does not respond by 1 g/dL in 4 weeks, the dose may be increased by 25%.

138. B: This study compared three-times-a-week and six-times-a-week in-center dialysis for two groups of 120–125 patients with chronic kidney disease. The results were published after a 12-month follow-up. Adherence in the six-times-a-week group was slightly less, averaging five times a week. Clearances (weekly *Kt/V*) were higher in the six-times-a-week group, and there was a 30%–40% reduction in two endpoints: death and left ventricular mass as measured by cardiac magnetic resonance imaging. There was also better control of hypertension and hyperphosphatemia in the more frequent dialysis group. There was no difference in depression, cognitive function, serum albumin level, or the need for erythropoiesis-stimulating agents. Vascular access, as might be expected, had more problems in the six-times-a-week group. One reviewing nephrology expert feels that a three-times-a-week, 3–4-hour dialysis schedule is not enough for many patients, but problems with adherence to schedules, adequate time and space at the center, and vascular access must be considered.

139. A: The structure of the nephron consists of a glomerulus and a renal tubule that connects to a collecting duct. Each kidney has about 1,000,000 nephrons. They consist of a glomerulus, proximal (descending) convoluted tubule, loop of Henle, and distal convoluted (ascending) tubule that connects to a collecting duct. The normal glomerular filtration rate is about 125 mL/min, which totals about 180 L/d. Glomerulae are tangled beds of capillaries held together by a membrane called Bowman's capsule. Blood is supplied to the glomerulus by the renal artery and an afferent arteriole and conducted away by an efferent arteriole. Nephrons are present in the renal cortex, but tubules descend into the medulla.

140. D: Acute tubular necrosis refers to an acute ischemic (lack of oxygen) injury to the renal tubules and is the leading cause of acute renal failure in hospitalized patients. Causes include blood transfusion reactions, muscle injury (rhabdomyolysis), shock, hypotension, and a variety of drugs and chemical agents. Examples of the latter are certain radiographic contrast media, aminoglycoside antibiotics, antifungal agents, and antineoplastic agents, such as certain platinum compounds. Liver disease or diabetic nephropathy may enhance susceptibility to this disorder.

While many patients recover total or partial renal function, some patients progress to chronic renal failure. Diminished (oliguria) or no (anuria) urine output may occur along with edema and symptoms of uremia. Many of these patients undergo hemodialysis to sustain them until renal function recovers or chronic renal failure ensues and persistent hemodialysis or renal transplantation is done.

141. C: The numerical formula Kt/V represents a number used to quantify adequacy of hemodialysis or peritoneal dialysis. K is the urea clearance of the dialyzer, t is the time of dialysis, and V is the volume of distribution of urea, approximately equal to the patient's total body water. The latter is usually calculated as 0.6 times patient weight in kilograms. Since K is in mL/min, t is in minutes, and V is in mL, the final dimension value cancels out to a dimensionless number. The Kt/V target recommended by the National Kidney Foundation is 1.3 for hemodialysis so that at least a prescription for 1.2 is reached. As an example, a 70-K patient, using a dialyzer with a K of 215 mL/min, a dialysis time of 4 hours (240 min), and a total body water of (70 K x 0.6 = 42 liters) or 42,000 mL, Kt/V is (215)(240)/42,000 = 1.23.

142. A: Fluid is removed from the blood and into the dialysate by ultrafiltration during hemodialysis. Diffusion decreases the solute concentration of the blood so that when the blood is recirculated into the patient, the higher solute concentration in cells and tissues gains fluid by osmosis, and blood volume is reduced. This reduction may cause hypotension and related symptoms. If sodium is added to the dialysate, it will diffuse into the blood and raise its osmotic pressure. This then draws water from the cells and tissues into the blood; the water is then removed during dialysis by the ultrafiltration pressure. The dialysate sodium concentration is often lowered toward the end of dialysis to allow the extra sodium to diffuse out of the blood.

143. B: Most complications for dialysis patients arise from vascular access problems. This may be due to inadequate blood supply from the access, thrombosis, or infection of the fistula or shunt. Poor cannulation may also play a role. These problems usually require a surgical revision or replacement of the access type, often with a temporary central venous catheter. According to statistics, 25%–50% of all hemodialysis patient hospitalizations are due to vascular access problems. This adds considerably to the cost of treatment. A dialysis session that is too long is unlikely to cause major problems, and mistaken prescriptions are rare since many of today's instructions are computer generated. Dietary indiscretions do occur but usually can be corrected with medication, change in dialysis formula, and duration or resumption of a proper diet.

144. C: Sterile techniques are used to protect patients from infection from other patients and from dialysis staff. Similarly, the reverse is also true for patients who have an infection. Bacteria and other microorganisms are easily transferred to patients from other individuals or surfaces. It should be noted that many patients undergoing dialysis are diabetic or immunosuppressed, rendering them at an increased risk for infectious disease. Hand washing is the single most important step in infection control. Soap and water or alcohol-based gels are satisfactory, but the former is preferred if hands are visibly dirty. Hands should be wet, and all surfaces rubbed vigorously with soap for at least 15 seconds, dried with a paper towel, and the towel used to shut off the faucet. Sterile gloves, surgical mask, and surgical gown may then be used as needed. Washing hands and donning fresh sterile gloves after a procedure or between patients constitute the best practice.

145. D: The environment around dialysis machines and equipment should be kept clean and often sterile. Note that patients bring in items, such as food or drink, that may be stored but never in the same refrigerator or cabinet as blood or tissue fluid samples or intravenous fluid containers. Patient reading material must also be considered a source of infection and be disposed of appropriately. All exterior surfaces, including the chair, bed, or counters at a station between patients should be cleaned. All pressure transducer protectors and cap dialyzer ports should be changed between patients, and used dialyzers and tubing should be put into leak-proof containers. Reprocessing used dialyzers ideally should be done in a separate room. Blood spills should be cleaned with bleach. Common equipment carts or medication trays should not be used; they should be delegated to a specific patient or washed between patients.

146. A: The nephrologist in charge of the patient to receive dialysis will provide a prescription, describing a variety of parameters for the dialysis. This specifies the length and frequency of dialysis, the specific dialyzer to use (brand, model, and size), the composition of the dialysate, the dose and mode of administration of heparin to be given, blood and dialysate flow rates, and ultrafiltration parameters. In addition, new or changes in continuing medication prescriptions may be included. Certain standard procedures, such as patient positioning, access cannulation, vital signs, patient weight, and charting details may not be specified if there is no departure from routine protocol.

147. B: Two major compatibility factors are considered in assessing suitable donors for a particular patient. Tissue typing analyzes the human leukocyte antigen (HLA) [genetically determined antigens on white blood cells] to see if they match the potential recipient. While there are over 100 of these antigens, some are more important in transplant rejection. Usually six are considered (e.g., HLA-1, HLA-B8). In families with the same mother and father, the children inherit one-half of his or her antigens from each parent. Thus, four possible combinations of antigens are possible, and there is a 25% chance that there will be a match, and a 25% chance that there will be no match at all. There is a 50% chance that there will be three out four antigen matches between brothers and sisters. A six-out-of-six antigen match is best for the success of the transplant, but lesser matches may be successful. Blood groups should also be matched, but people with type O (universal donors) may donate to all of those with the four major blood groups (O, A, B, AB).

148. C: Chronic kidney disease is often categorized clinically by the glomerular filtration rate (GFR), usually measured by the creatinine clearance and adjusted to the body surface area (e.g., 100 mL/min/1.73 m²). Stage 1 patients who have a GFR over 90 mL/min rarely have symptoms. Stage 2 patients have a GFR in the 60–89 mL/min and may have mild symptoms. Patients with a GFR in the 30–59 mL/min usually show systemic symptoms, abnormal calcium and phosphate levels, edema. and hypertension and are in the stage 3 category. Stage 4 patients with a GFR in the 15–29 mL/min range may be considered for dialysis or transplantation, and stage 5 (GFR less than 15 mL/min) is always an indication for dialysis.

149. A: Numerous physicians and bioengineers have played important roles in developing modern dialysis and its associated techniques. The first use of dialysis with a crude rotating drum and use of sausage casing is credited to Willem J. Kolff, MD, a Dutch physician, in 1943. Fresh arteries and veins were used so there was a limitation on the duration of treatment. Mostly it was used for patients who were expected to recover kidney function. Belding H. Scribner, MD, and associates developed the external shunt blood access in 1960 so that patients with chronic renal failure could be treated. The arteriovenous fistula developed by James A. Cimino, MD, in 1966 reduced clotting and infection problems since native vessels were attached to each other, and the connection was entirely within the arm. Gregory House, MD, was a famous otologist and ear surgeon (or a TV doctor with a nasty disposition) who did not play a role in dialysis development.

150. D: Renal osteodystrophy refers to the bone demineralization seen in chronic kidney disease. It may be divided into high- or low-bone turnover types. Symptoms may be bone or joint pain, fractures, or bone deformation. Blood tests usually show a low-calcium and high-phosphate levels since the diseased kidney is unable to excrete phosphate. Calcitriol, the active form of vitamin D, is low, which contributes to poor absorption of calcium. The parathyroid hormone is elevated due to low-calcium levels that stimulate the parathyroid glands so that this disorder is associated with secondary hyperparathyroidism. Calcium and vitamin D supplements, phosphate binders, and hemodialysis are all indicated. Renal transplantation may be curative.

Additional Bonus Material

Due to our efforts to try to keep this book to a manageable length, we've created a link that will give you access to all of your additional bonus material:

mometrix.com/bonus948/certhemotech

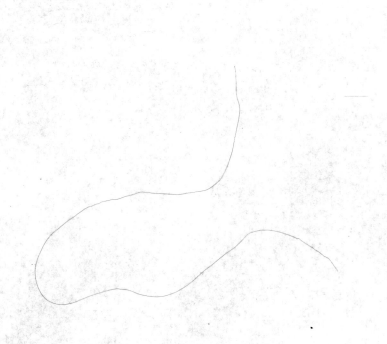